I Have
Something
to Tell You

I Have Something to Tell You

A Memoir

Regan Hofmann

ATRIA BOOKS

New York   London   Toronto   Sydney

ATRIA BOOKS
A Division of Simon & Schuster, Inc.
1230 Avenue of the Americas
New York, NY 10020

First Atria Books hardcover edition September 2009

ATRIA BOOKS and colophon are trademarks of Simon & Schuster, Inc.

For information about special discounts for bulk purchases, please contact Simon & Schuster Special Sales at 1-866-506-1949 or business@simonandschuster.com.

The Simon & Schuster Speakers Bureau can bring authors to your live event. For more information or to book an event contact the Simon & Schuster Speakers Bureau at 1-866-248-3049 or visit our website at www.simonspeakers.com.

Designed by Jill Putorti

Manufactured in the United States of America

10   9   8   7   6   5   4   3   2   1

Library of Congress Cataloging-in-Publication Data
Hofmann, Regan.
I have something to tell you : a memoir / by Regan Hofmann.—1st Atria Books hardcover ed.
    p. cm.
1. Hofmann, Regan. 2. AIDS (Disease)—Patients—United States—Biography. 3. AIDS activists—United States—Biography. 4. Editors—United States—Biography. I. Title.
RC606.55.H+A3 2009
362.196'97920092—dc22
[B]

2009013502

ISBN 978-1-4165-9859-6
ISBN 978-1-4391-0964-9 (ebook)

For my loving family, who saved my life.

To the memory of Jody, who changed it.

Your silence will not protect you.

—AUDRE LORDE

You can't start a fire worrying about
your little world falling apart.

—BRUCE SPRINGSTEEN,

FROM "DANCING IN THE DARK"

Silence = Death

—ACT UP SLOGAN, 1987

note to readers

This work is a memoir. It reflects the author's present recollections of her experiences over a period of years. Certain names, locations, and identifying characteristics have been changed, and certain individuals are composites. Dialogue and events have been re-created from memory and, in some cases, have been compressed to convey the substance of what was said or what occurred.

prologue

I am a walking biohazard—a heated container of deadly viral particles. I don't look sick. But I could kill you. I am part of a tribe of people bound by bad biology: misunderstood, deeply feared because of the human immunodeficiency virus I carry and bearing a crippling stigma that has long kept me silent.

Writing this is a bloodletting. My pen pierces a hematoma of shame that swelled until holding it in became too painful. This is how it had to happen: the pain of not telling became greater than the fear of what would happen if I told. When too much vital life force collects in an unnatural place it can't be contained. It turns fetid and festers—infecting the person who holds it in with a vicious disease. Eventually, it explodes outward.

The flood of relief following the sting when the secret is lanced is replaced by the awkwardness of staring at the mess the release has created. Will you look at that? Now what have you done? Who is going to clean it up? But ultimately, you are healed. The virus threatens death but stigma surely kills. Other people's fear and ignorance about what is nothing more than a retrovirus deny my dignity. And there is no point in living without that.

After all, what did I do?

Had sex without a condom.

For this, I should suffer and die, silent and alone?

I am no different from others who thought they were immune to HIV. We made the same choice; HIV just happened to be there when I made mine. The fact that I'm HIV-positive doesn't make me a bad person, just an unlucky one. But because many people don't understand this, I kept silent about my disease for fear that I would lose my friends, my job, my home, my sanity.

One of the worst symptoms of HIV is secrecy. If you get cancer? You can get help. Compassion. Love. Empathy. Praise for your heroism through the struggle. If you lose your hair, you get wigs. If you get HIV? You get secretive. Insular. Paranoid. Your life becomes a giant pretense so no one finds out you have this disease. You don't know what people will do for you because you are too afraid to tell them. You try desperately not to lose your mind. There are no wigs to cover up that loss.

When you have HIV, you are deadly, but not necessarily dying any faster than anyone else. You're maybe not even sick yet. But by being labeled terminal, you remind people of the reality we all share but would rather not face: that we are all going to die. You are a walking ad for the fragility of life. And people don't like to have their illusion of invincibility eroded. People fear people with HIV in part because we remind them that no one is immune to death.

Ten years is a long time to stay quiet—about anything. When the secret you won't share is that you're fighting for your life, time passes in a peculiar way. It's like you're living at hyper-speed weighted down to slow motion by the burden of your secrecy. The way your impending death rushes at you coupled with your efforts to make whatever life you have left last as long as possible makes you ache in parts of yourself that you never knew existed.

You burn the candle at both ends—and the middle—trying to suck the lifeblood out of each day because you understand that this could be your last day on earth. Once you believe that, everything changes.

For a decade, I harbored my secret, waiting for them to find the cure, waiting to be healed—by an acupuncturist, a faith healer, wheat grass, a miracle. By the divine intervention of Jesus, Yahweh, Allah, Buddha, Krishna—any god would do. I wanted to die any other way but from HIV.

I dreamed of purging the vile visitor from my bloodstream. I imagined getting my labs done and discovering that the virus was gone. I woke up each morning hoping that the daylight had scared the nightmare of HIV from my blood. But each day, it was still there, well after I'd showered, dressed and had my tea.

In time, I accepted that I was going to have to live with the virus peaceably or it would have a better shot at killing me. I inspected it by microscope, admiring its otherworldly beauty. I tried my best to appreciate its resilience and adaptability. While it repeatedly foiled research scientists' attempts to quell its replication, rather than resent its tenacity, I told myself that it was only doing what every living thing does: trying to survive everything that tries to kill it.

Eventually, I embraced the idea that HIV was here to stay. I told myself that if the virus was sticking around, I was, too.

Somehow, it got easier to live—though I was dying.

But nothing lessened my fear of being stigmatized.

It's hard to describe how I feel when I hear the word "AIDS" hissed under someone's breath like a cobra. AIDS rarely rolls off anyone's tongue. It's spit out with venom. AIDS! Blech, blech,

blech. Wipe the back of your hand against your mouth after you say it. Spit again just to make sure all traces of it are gone.

You have to tell yourself over and over that it's the virus that repulses people—not you.

For so many years, I waited to hear someone say "AIDS" the way we have learned to say breast or colon cancer. I hoped that since we'd evolved to a place where we could easily and politely speak of other diseases connected to sexual organs and parts of the body that make some people squeamish, we could learn to talk about AIDS in the same way.

I waited for a day when the pharmacist would call, "Hofmann?" and hand me my bags of hard-to-swallow but life-saving medicine without giving me a knowing wink that was one part curiosity (What's a nice girl like you doing in a situation like this?), one part better-you-than-me-babe and a dash of disgust.

But I waited in vain.

There were mornings when I worried whether it would be my last and I felt like I was dying and it would have been nice to call in sick, go and have a glass of wine with a friend and cry my pain out while she held on to me. There were so many times when I desperately wanted to tell the people around me that I needed help to get through feeling like I'd swallowed a hand grenade—after its pin had been pulled out.

Finally, when I couldn't bear the loneliness and fear any longer, I told the people closest to me—my sister and my parents—that I had HIV. Over the years, the secret crept out to a few more people such as my riding coach, several doctors and the men I considered dating. Mostly though, shame sealed my lips. I didn't tell a single friend for almost ten years.

Whenever I told others that I had HIV, they told me a secret. They lost the baby. They killed someone by accident. They would rather be a woman.

These moments of unexpected disclosure happened with people I knew well and people I didn't know at all. Sharing my HIV status seemed to compel others to unfurl their own deep truths. I wondered whether their doing so was an act of empathy, of commiseration intended to say, without saying, that they understood, that it was okay and that HIV was not the worst thing that can happen to a person. Or maybe it was easier for people to talk about their own horrors than to say something—anything—about a subject as scary as HIV.

Perhaps people realized that if I could admit that I had HIV, anything could be said. Just like that: you open your mouth and the worry of having your secret eat you alive is gone. It felt so good to let go of the burden of a thing that was heavier for having rarely been spoken. I told the truth and the terror ended.

Because no matter how dark your secret is, it gets lighter each time you tell it to someone else.

Though I revealed my status several times out of necessity, the thought of telling the wide world never occurred to me. I never told anyone about what it's *really* like to live with HIV as a young, single American woman. Because I didn't want others to worry about me. Because I didn't want to burden them with the truth. And because I was too afraid of how they would judge me.

Until now.

WINTER 1996–FALL 1997

CHAPTER
one

I spent the last carefree moments of my life swimming with dolphins. My mom had sponsored dolphins on behalf of both my younger sister Tracy and me, and given them to us as Christmas presents. We unwrapped flat boxes containing pictures of the smiling, slate-colored marine mammals and stared, bewildered, until my mom pointed out that there was something beneath the photos—a plane ticket. The other part of her gift was to take the three of us to Florida to see the bottle-nosed creatures in person. Our dolphins lived at a sanctuary that allowed people to visit; their survival depended, in part, on the generosity of people like my mom. I loved the idea of having my own dolphin.

Ever since I was a small child, I have been obsessed with animals. My mom and I have spent a fortune on food and vet care for feral and misplaced cats, dogs, ewes, hawks, raccoons and horses who rarely understood the help we provided—as a result, we often got bitten, scratched, pecked or kicked while trying to save their lives. We've learned that it is safer to fulfill our urge to rescue animals by financially supporting wildlife from afar and letting the pros handle things. There is a manatee and a timber wolf living the high life somewhere thanks to my hard-earned dollar. But, God help me if a wounded, dazed raccoon stumbles down the road in front of my car. I'm putting on the oven mitts I carry in my trunk (especially for situations like that) and I'm going to get my furry friend into a box (also always in my car, just in case) and I'm going to take him to the wildlife center, rabies be damned.

One time, I collected a vulture with a broken wing. He lay quietly on a blanket on my back seat, until a squirrel ran out in front of me. I jammed on the brakes and the vulture tried to keep his balance by flapping his good wing—a move that somehow tossed him into the passenger seat. A guy in a pickup truck next to me at a red light looked at my winged copilot with his mouth agape. I guess I did look a little crazy with the giant, black, flesh-eating bird sitting quietly beside me, but I don't discriminate when it comes to the kinds of things I will try to save. Worms, bugs, bats, rats, snakes, weasels and raptors all deserve to live, too. After all, a rat is just a squirrel with no fur on its tail. Whether one is cute and the other is vermin depends entirely on how you look at things.

Several months after our dolphins were given to us, my mom, sister and I found ourselves on different planes, my mom from New Jersey, Tracy from Washington, DC, and me from Atlanta, traveling to a land of sunlight and sand to see them.

We met at the Miami airport in a flurry of giddy hugs and collected our rental car. My mother careened with uncharacteristic speed out of the airport piloting the Dodge Intrepid over an endless series of little bridges linking the archipelago in the

Gulf Stream toward Grassy Key—home of the Dolphin Research Center.

We hurtled between wide swaths of blue sea, over hump after hump of paved arches as if we were tracing the outline of the back of a Brachiosaurus. The name of our car—the Intrepid—perfectly characterized our journey. None of us was sure where we were going next in our lives, but we were going there full throttle. My sister, who was then twenty-six, was dating her husband-to-be Josh and studying law in DC. I was twenty-eight, working as a freelance writer and recovering from a heartbreaking divorce. Andrew—my dashingly handsome, sweet first husband—and I had split up a mere eleven months after getting married in the spring of 1994. During our marriage, weekend after weekend, we woke up on Saturday mornings wanting to do profoundly different things. Andrew wanted to play golf and have me wait for him in a crisply pleated tennis skirt at the country club's "nineteenth hole"; I wanted to search the woods in camouflage pants, looking for animal bones, antlers, turtle shells, feathers and nests to add to my collection of natural curiosities that I'd started years ago.

As a child I spied a bleached cow skull at the edge of the woods while riding around a golf course in the cart with my dad. We'd picked it up, and my dad, who painted as a hobby to unwind from days of working as a CEO, placed it on the kitchen table and spent weeks integrating its form into his various watercolor landscapes. Bones had always been things of beauty to me; to Andrew, they were dirty and strange.

Sadly, Andrew and I didn't realize we were irreconcilably different until we were already married. He wanted me to make the homemade breakfasts he'd never had as a child; I never cooked, preferring stacks of syrup-slathered silver dollar pancakes at IHOP. I would talk endlessly and loudly about my feelings; he would listen, saying little in response. Not that you could ever reduce three years of love to pancakes and how we expressed ourselves, but these things pointed to fundamentally different ways that we moved through the world, ways that would not allow us to do that side by side unless one of us changed who we were. And we both liked who we were. We just hadn't known ourselves, or been able to express who we were clearly enough to the other before we decided to spend the rest of our lives together. We parted brokenheartedly as friends.

As my mom, Tracy and I hurtled that day through the Keys, I was still reeling from the double shock of marrying such a seemingly perfect man who was so perfectly wrong for me and the notion that I was starting my whole life over at twenty-eight—so soon after I thought I'd figured it all out.

I briefly dated one man, Antonio, post-divorce, but had called off our relationship just months after it began when it was clear that I was unready to give my heart to someone new.

My mother was married to a man named Frank, whom she married the same year Andrew and I did, two years after her divorce from my father. My parents, who had been married twenty-seven years, split up when I was twenty-five. Subconsciously, I thought that my marriage to Andrew might help bring everyone back together. Little did I know that the fabric of even the most tightly knit families runs the risk of being torn to shreds by the stress and the expense of orchestrating a black-tie wedding for hundreds of people. And that when a marriage is over, the canned happiness of a party will never glue it back together.

My mom, my sister and I had all recently made choices that changed our lives forever, and we were still in that stage between making those choices and finding out whether or not they were the right ones. And so, we were filled with a certain lightness—amplified by being three grown women on the loose for a long weekend with nothing to do but sit in the sun, eat, drink rum, talk and play with dolphins.

My mother had uncharacteristically tied her shoulder-length dark brown hair back in a loose ponytail with a scarf. Normally, it fell about her shoulders in soft chocolate curls. I wondered if she'd left her hot rollers behind. I hoped so. I had almost never seen my mother's thick, dark wavy hair uncurled. As a young girl, I used to love going in to kiss her good night after she'd emerged from the shower, fresh and warm, wrapped always in a bathrobe that felt like a stuffed animal. She would twist her wet hair into a Carmen-Miranda-esque pile of terry cloth on her head, the weight of which pulled the corners of her eyes up exotically. By the next morning, her dark mane was inevitably blown dry and curled. She rarely went out in public without looking like a movie star. Not that she had to try to look like one. Because of her beautiful bone structure and thick cascade of hair, a quick swipe of her frosted coral lipstick was all she needed to look glamorous. It seemed a promising forecast of fun for our Florida girls' weekend that my mom had let down her hair.

As we sped southward down the highway, I noticed that Tracy, who is two and a half years younger than I am but whose elegant and stoic queen-mother-like disposition makes everyone think she's older, also seemed atypically relaxed. She wore a scoop-necked tank top, which exposed more of the delicate winter-white skin of her décolletage than she typically allowed. I worried that the sun would make mincemeat of her skin, but knowing her, she'd already slathered herself in SPF 40s—just in case a ray of sun crawled in through the tinted glass of the car.

I'd made a mixed tape for our journey with a little Johnny Cash, some Elvis and a lot of Grateful Dead. As we drove, I stuck my hand out the window and let the wind slide hot and dry down the underside of my arm into my loose sundress. I kicked off my shoes and pulled the ponytail holder from my shoulder-length blond hair; the breeze blew away the stress of a long winter. My mom turned the radio up and we all belted out "Good Lovin' " at the top of our out-of tune voices. Laughing at how awful we sounded, I was reminded of my grandfather saying, "If all the birds in the forest with bad voices stopped singing the woods would be a very quiet place." There was something to that; together, we sounded fine.

After nearly two hours of driving and a stop at the Shell Man (where I added to my collection of natural curios with the purchase of a red Bahamian starfish, curls of conchs that replayed the ocean's pounding roar in my ear and a giant nautilus polished shiny by the tumbling waves—ironically, the symbol of eternal life), we arrived at the Dolphin Research Center ready, as their website suggested, to "get wet with a dolphin."

The center had rehabilitated the original Flipper (the inspiration for the movie), who'd famously gotten stuck in a fisherman's net, and befriended the man who saved him. Since then, the center has rescued, studied and advocated on behalf of all species of marine mammals. Its work was instrumental in stopping the slaughter of whales.

I was highly skeptical that I'd meet my actual dolphin (would I be able to recognize her from her picture, anyway?) but the trainers at the Dolphin Research Center promised us that we would be personally thanked by our dolphins for my mother's generous donation. After registering, we went to our rooms and eventually reemerged—dressed in bathing suits and pareos, ready for orientation. In a classroom made of several wooden benches under a thatched roof, we listened to a sun-cured man in a big-brimmed hat and a zinc-oxided nose describe the history of dolphin rescue and research.

He told us how, when the hurricanes came, the staff lowered the underwater chain-link fences that formed the dolphins' paddocks so they could swim to safety in the open ocean. He said the dolphins almost always came back. I felt much better knowing that the dolphins my mom was supporting were semiwild. I would not want her to endow dolphins kept in chlorined captivity in touristy resorts forced to swim with screaming children or get no fish for dinner. The rule at the DRC was that it was up to the dolphin, not the guest, whether or not there would be swimming that day.

Using a large plastic facsimile of a male dolphin, the trainer showed us where it was safe to stroke the dolphin and where it was ill advised to do so; the swipe of a human hand on the wrong part of the dolphin's anatomy could arouse an affection that could be deadly. We nodded solemnly and promised to keep our hands above the water.

Anyone who doubts the intelligence of dolphins needs only to see the complexity of their call signs to understand their brainpower. The trainers summon the dolphins to the surface with large, white, intricate symbols made out of wood, fastened to the end of long poles they dip into the water. As my mom, Tracy and I stood breathlessly on the AstroTurf–covered dock in our bathing suits, a trainer lowered one of the giant swizzle sticks into the water and waved it about—nothing. He waited a bit and then, switching sticks, plunged another under the surface of the lagoon. Suddenly, I saw the dark blur of a dolphin twenty feet away. He jetted for the surface and erupted with a comical grin on his face, landing on his back in the wake of his own splash, chattering his triangular teeth, begging for fish.

We applauded. I have no idea why, but I clapped my hands together like a small child at the sight of this magnificent creature who stared back at us with curiosity and penetrating intelligence. There is something unnerving about looking into the eyes of a beast so attuned to nature's subtleties that it can sense a hurricane hours before the most sophisticated technology can detect the same atmospheric disturbance.

One by one, we slid into the sea to play with the dolphins. At the trainer's suggestion, I twirled around while treading water, splashing my hands on the gray-green lagoon. On the trainer's command, the dolphin attempted to copy me. He stood up on his tail and spun in circles, smacking the water with his fins.

The dolphins can sense things we can't. If you're scared, they swim slowly. If you're brave, they speed up. They refused to pull one young woman, trying repeatedly to take her back to shore. The dolphin trainer asked if she was sick. She said no. The next day, she shared with us what the dolphins had perceived—that she was newly pregnant.

When it was my turn for my favorite game, the "dorsal pull," I swam out to the middle of the lagoon and spread my arms. I felt the pair of 500-pound dolphins beneath me, stirring the water with their massive bodies, which move as a single muscle. As they rose from the deep in tandem, I grabbed hold of their dorsal fins tightly; they pulled me across the water with an exhilarating jerk. I let my legs go limp; don't try to swim, the instructor had said. Just go with their flow. They circled around and around, taking me farther out than they had the others. I laughed out loud, my mouth filling with foamy seawater. They seemed to know I was having the time of my life. Maybe they knew that it was the last time I would ever feel this free.

* * *

I first discovered the lump while I was waiting on the dock for my second turn to swim. I dropped my arm to swat a sand fly on my thigh and the inside of my wrist brushed against a bump the size of half a golf ball nestled in the groove where my leg met my body. I pressed on it. It didn't hurt. It was just unsightly. I looked over my shoulder for Tracy, wanting to show it to her, but she was out in the water, being swept up by the dolphins. When she returned to the dock, I showed the bump to her and my mom; neither of them seemed alarmed.

The thought that something was threatening my life never occurred to me. For the rest of the weekend, my mom and Tracy and I played with the dolphins, flew across the glassy surface of the lagoon on wave runners and added rum floaters to our piña coladas at dinner, singing along with the acoustic guitarist who serenaded us at the water's edge as the sun sank into the sea.

When it was time to go, we vowed to make a yearly ritual of our pilgrimage.

When I got home to Atlanta, the lump in my groin still hadn't gone away, so I went to my doctor and showed it to him. He seemed as unconcerned as my mom and sister. He said it could be mono, or cat scratch disease, and proposed a litany of tests, including one for HIV just to be safe; I barely paid attention when I signed the waiver for the HIV test. I'd been tested throughout my life and didn't think there was any way I could have been exposed to the virus.

Even when they called me a week later to say that the results of my blood work were inconclusive and that I'd need to come back in to have more blood drawn I wasn't worried. On the phone, the nurse explained they needed to do some follow-up test, but that she didn't know why.

At the doctor's I sat in an exam room, patiently reading. After twenty minutes, a nurse came in, told me my doctor was running late and asked, "Do you mind waiting in the doctor's private office? We need this room to examine another patient."

That should have been my first clue that something was awry. Why not just send me back to the waiting room? But thinking I had no reason for concern, I said, "No problem," and followed her down the hallway to my doctor's office. The nurse opened the door and offered me a seat in a big, black, leather La-Z-Boy recliner in front of an oversized TV.

"Can I get you something to drink?" she offered.

If I'd known what was coming, I would have asked for tequila. Instead, I asked for a Diet Coke.

"So, this is what my doctor does while I'm waiting for him, endlessly," I joked, pointing at the humongous TV set. She smiled professionally and showed me how to use the control wand to adjust the angle of the chair and to turn on the different massage modes.

There was a moment when it seemed a little strange—me, wiggling away in this huge recliner, watching *The Jerry Springer Show* in my doctor's private space—but I quelled the instinct to listen to the sudden small ache deep in my stomach. Had I been a dolphin, feral and free, I would have left the scene that was about to unfold. But as a human trained to ignore nature's most obvious signs, I just sat there, relaxed. Any subconscious knowledge I might have had that something was wrong was overridden by the perpetual optimism that was, until then, part of my emotional composition.

I'd been carefully conditioned to think that if I followed the laws of society, I'd be protected—except from the things that no one could ever be protected from, like serial killers, errant asteroids and plagues. The illusion of control had been drilled into me at places like the Barclay ballroom dance classes in my hometown of Princeton, where at the age of thirteen, I first clutched the hands of young men through the safety of white cotton gloves; the freezing chop of the Connecticut River at dawn, where I stroked the eight-woman varsity crew for Trinity College; and the sand arena of my British, Olympian riding coach, Carol. As long as I did the right thing, my instructors taught me, I would be safe.

I moved the chair around, watching the emotionally torn-up people on *Jerry Springer* swing wildly at each other as plainclothes policemen tried to restrain them. I was astonished that people could hurt badly enough to be oblivious to humiliating themselves on national television.

I wish I could say I was reprimanding myself for watching the misfortune of others, when the door banged opened and a squadron of people in white lab coats walked into the room. But the truth is, I was thinking how glad I was to have been born and raised in a world far, far away from that of *Jerry Springer*'s guests. And then, suddenly, I wasn't merely watching other people's lives fall apart on daytime television; I was smack dab in the middle of my own *Jerry Springer* moment.

I knew from the doctors' faces, and their number, that whatever it was, it was bad. Had I contracted some rare tropical disease from the dolphins? Was the man on the far left, who was not my doctor, from the government? Were they going to quarantine me? Would I get to make some phone calls? I started to feel as if I were in a sci-fi movie. I thought about those films where people get sucked unwillingly into medical experiments and awaken in water-filled tanks with strange plugs in their bodies.

My doctor coughed nervously and one of the nurses switched a file folder that was clamped beneath one elbow to the other. As she whisked the folder across her body, a giant gold liquid-filled syringe fell out. It stuck in the carpet, swaying back and forth on its point—like a sinister metronome, counting away the last seconds of my innocence.

As soon as I saw the syringe, I knew something terrible was about to happen.

"Whatever it is," I said to the group dressed forebodingly in white in front of me, "however bad it is, please do not stick that in me."

The needle was long enough to penetrate through clothes, fat and muscle, deep inside a body where the sedative would work immediately. It was strong enough not to break during the thrashing of a disturbed soul.

No one looked at me while the doctor told me the news. He turned off the TV, cleared his throat and said, "I don't know how to tell you this, so I'm just going to tell you. Your blood work shows that you are HIV-positive. I am so sorry."

I took several half breaths. "I don't have cat scratch disease?" I asked, frantically hoping he would say, "Oh, did I say HIV? I meant cat scratch disease."

"No, I'm afraid not," he said gently, his tired eyes searching my face.

"Turn it off. Please, turn this chair off," I said, fumbling with the control wand, trying to get the chair to stop vibrating. So this is why they brought me in here: to relax me before telling me the news. A nurse came over and pressed a button on the control wand and the shaking stopped.

How long, I wondered, is long enough to jiggle before you're relaxed enough to be told you're dying? Twenty minutes? An hour? A day? The rest of your life, what's left of it? Is a gentle lower lumbar massage really going to calm your pounding heart so that it does not splinter your ribs? I looked at them looking at me; we were all speechless. I knew a new kind of quiet—one caused by a silence that falls when there is only one person in the room who should speak and that person can't say a word. I couldn't even grunt. The weight of all the unuttered answers to the questions ricocheting around my head intensified the silence.

It just couldn't be. I'd been so careful. Prudish, even. I'd never used IV drugs and I'd almost always used a condom. My mind spun over the faces of my past partners—but I'd been fine and they'd been fine and were all healthy and I was healthy except for this virus now. It was so strange: I looked perfectly okay, felt perfectly okay, and yet was in the midst of a life-or-death battle with a virus that would soon wither me like a plant with no roots.

I couldn't move. My body felt two-dimensional. I closed my eyes. The three letters floated around on the black insides of my closed eyelids, swirling, connecting, disconnecting and reconnecting in various triumvirates—VIH, IVH, HVI, HIV—like a maniacal bowl of Alpha-Bits cereal.

My mind exploded in every direction: great and unbearable fear at the notion of a slow, humiliating, painful death; grief so penetrating it felt like the air had been let out of my soul; ecstasy that I was free of everything I never wanted to do; the feeling that all was very, very wrong inside of me and a weird certainty that I wasn't going to die from this.

"Turn it back on," I said. "Please, turn the chair on."

The nurse came bumbling toward me again.

"Here," I said, handing her the control. She stabbed at the buttons with her square-tipped, ruby-colored nails, happy to have something else to concentrate on besides my face. I wasn't crying. Didn't look scared. Wasn't angry. Because I was in lobotomizing shock. The kind I imagine passengers experience when the airline captain comes on the PA system and says, "That's it, folks. I'm sorry. There's nothing else I can do. God bless and keep you. Over and out." I've always liked to believe that when you really know something unspeakably horrible is about to happen, your mind saves itself, shutting down to avoid having to register what it knows is coming.

Maybe they were wrong. Maybe there had been a mistake. Perhaps I was going to make history as the first person diagnosed with HIV for whom both vials of blood had been accidentally switched in the lab. They *had* to be wrong. People don't die from disease at twenty-eight. People who are in their late twenties die in a flash, a crash, an OD, a shot. They don't have time to think about it. No one faces death on a day when cream-white clouds swirl in the blue tea of the sky. Death comes on dark nights, the wind undressing the trees, howling in complaint of their bony nakedness. It comes to people left alone in a pool of bodily fluid on the roof of an abandoned parking garage, or in a bed after months of prolonged, body-withering sickness, or in an explosion of light and glass and metal and sound. People don't die on beautiful days when the promise of a party brightens the drudgery of a work day, drawing the neighbors together to share cheer, the ice in their crystal tumblers tinkling like tiny bells.

My neighbor's party. Can you imagine their faces when I called? "Hi, listen, it's Regan. I was just diagnosed as terminally ill this afternoon and I don't think I'll be able to join you after all. I hope you understand. Would you like me to drop off the brownies anyway?" It seemed unthinkable that death could intrude so rudely and prematurely into my nicely planned life.

I looked at the doctor, and asked, "How long? How long do I have to live?"

"I don't know," he said. "A year. Maybe two. HIV progresses much more quickly in women. Unless you can identify when you might have gotten it, it's hard to guess."

"One year!? How will you know if it's one year or two?" I asked desperately.

"We'll test you again soon. We'll also see how your viral load changes over time."

"What about kids?" I asked in a tiny, breathless voice.

"No," the doctor said.

"Sex?" I whispered.

"Probably not a good idea," he said.

As if anyone would ever want to get near me now.

The nurses flanking the doctor looked like altar boys: dressed in white, standing at rapt attention, well rehearsed in the proceedings, waiting patiently for their cue to act. I wondered if they were religious, and if so, if they were praying for me.

"How are you doing?" the nurse asked. She pointed to the syringe still stuck in the carpet. It had stopped swaying. Time was up. "You want some help? I could just give you a little bit. It might make things . . . easier," she said.

"No," I blurted out. I wanted my head clear to think.

I was going to die, sexless for the rest of my life, without the ability to leave behind a legacy in the form of a child. Not only was I going to have to tell my mother, father and sister that they would lose their daughter and sister, I couldn't even give them a part of me to hold on to after I was gone.

The reality that I had HIV moved slowly through my mind. The idea was as easily digestible as a large chunk of metal. It just couldn't be. What about all my friends who'd been so much wilder? They were okay. Why wasn't I? All that sex I'd not had for the sake of good health and propriety and self-respect and this was what I had to show for it? A deadly STD?

My mind wheeled like a kite in a crosswind. Who had done this to me? I thought about my past boyfriends. Andrew, my ex-husband. Antonio, my most recent ex-boyfriend. We had broken up several months ago; how was I going to tell him? I worried about everything at once: that he gave it to me; that I gave it to him; that even though the results of my past HIV tests indicated otherwise, that I'd had it a long time and had given it to others, too; that he would kill me if I'd given it to him; that he would kill himself when I told him I had it; that I would kill him if he'd given it to me; that I'd kill myself for getting it; that I would die.

I knew Antonio for a year before we dated; he seemed so clean and safe. He had a nice family. He sang to me and let me drive the boat with his arms wrapped protectively around my shoulders when we went waterskiing on a nearby lake. He washed my hair, tenderly, with a sponge and a bucket at the barn when the power was out after a thunderstorm. It was hard to believe he had the capacity, or intent, to kill me.

"Do you have someone to go to?" the doctor asked.

Who could I go to with this? But I said anyway, "Yes, I have someone."

"I'm giving you a prescription for some medicine to take away any anxiety you might feel. Don't be afraid to take it. I'm also giving you a phone number for an infectious disease doctor and a counselor who specializes in these kinds of things," he said.

Ah, *these* kinds of things. He handed me small slips of paper with phone numbers and the prescription. I noticed he put down a quantity of only six pills. Not enough to end it.

On the way out of the doctor's office, they asked me to pay my bill. They should not do this. Perhaps they bill you on the spot because they worry you will go home and blow your brains out. In case you're wondering, they charge you $250 to tell you you are dying.

CHAPTER
two

Somehow, I managed to find my car, get to the drugstore, fill my extremely disappointing prescription and drive home.

When I got there, I lay on the sofa, watching the sun drag the day down from the sky. I looked around my apartment seeing my furniture and paintings and stuff as if it all belonged to someone else. I couldn't even bear to go into my bedroom—the mosquito-net-encased bed with the sheets still tangled from the night before made me think of sex and how HIV had entered my body. I lay on a mint-green brocade couch I had pulled from the curb and had intended to reupholster but, disheartened after my divorce, never got around to it. The clock read six. The whole day had slipped away. Suddenly, I realized I was hungry. It felt strange to feel my body. Since leaving the doctor's office, it was as if my mind had done everything it could to separate itself from my infested little self.

I uncorked some Chardonnay, poured the yellow liquid into a red wine glass the size of a small fishbowl and put on some Prince. I decided to make pasta.

Watching the water bubble in the pot while the sauce percolated, the totality of my transformation began to emerge. There was something oddly exhilarating about playing the lead role in a tragedy of this proportion. My days on the planet were numbered. I wondered if I was being taken away because I had something more important to do somewhere else—or in another lifetime. I poured the scarlet sauce over a pile of elbow macaroni that looked like tiny bones and ate voraciously, astounded at the complexities of the smells and flavors I had never noticed before in Prego. I licked the bowl—something I usually didn't allow myself to do. Manners had been drilled so indelibly into me that even when I yawned while driving alone in my car, I covered my mouth. The realization that I didn't care anymore, that I could do anything I wanted from here on in, was the first happy thought I'd had since my diagnosis. Buoyed slightly by the thought of my freedom from obligation, I decided to shower, wondering whether the sensory overload my current state of mind was affording me would continue under the water.

I turned on the faucet and took off my clothes. I looked at my naked self in the mirror. A ghost of me—terrifyingly terrified—stared back. My face still wore the expression it had when they'd shared the news. My eyes looked like two raisins dropped in the snow.

Anger I'd suppressed for hours welled in my throat, rising like a regurgitated ball of steel wool. A scream originated in some dark corner of myself I didn't know existed, erupting from my mouth while my hands slapped at the walls of the bathroom as if controlled by the jerking of some crazed puppeteer in time to the staccato beat of my bare feet stomping the floor. My hands pounded the image of my stupid, filthy, unforgivable self in the mirror while my eyes reeled wildly around, looking for something to hold on to. Recoiling from my reflection and stepping into the cascade of scalding water, I grabbed the shower curtain with both hands, yanking and tearing and pulling and stretching until it popped free from its wire rings, falling in a heap on top of me. Hot drops of water lanced my naked back as burning rivulets streaked my face sliding, as I did, to the floor, wrapping myself in the wet plastic, laying my head on the steaming porcelain.

Disintegration. Disgrace. Denial. Darkness. Dying. Death. Dead. How could I have let this happen to me?

I finally got up and had the courage to look at myself in the cracked mirror; beads of condensation crawled down its surface. My face looked like it was melting. I forced my legs to carry me from the bathroom to my bedroom, and fell face down on my bed. The thought that consumed me as I lay there was that HIV hadn't just *happened* to me. Someone had *given* it to me, and I had to find out who it was. Just thinking about the phone calls I'd have to make was enough to make my stomach convulse. I was so afraid to tell anyone I'd been with, but as much as I didn't want to face the men I'd been with, I knew I couldn't let them nor the women they'd been with die.

Who had given this to me?

I'd been with Andrew exclusively for two years prior to our getting married. We had both gotten HIV tests before the wedding, so I knew neither of us brought HIV into the marriage. Had he cheated on me and given it to me during our marriage? And Antonio? Because I was on birth control, and because I had asked him whether he'd ever used IV drugs or been with sex workers or a man and he said "no" on all counts, we'd not used a condom. I really didn't think I was at risk. I had been totally paranoid about getting an STD in my early twenties, but by my late twenties, I didn't think about it as much—and I'd never heard of a woman who'd gotten HIV from unprotected sex with a straight man.

Just before bed, I poured a glass of water and opened the little plastic container of my AIDS meds. In addition to the prescription, for antianxiety pills, my doctor had also prescribed antiretroviral medicine to fight the HIV. I dumped the blue-and-white pills into my hand, staring at the shiny gel caps, remembering what the doctor had told me: "They won't cure you, or stop the HIV from destroying your immune system. But they may buy you some more time by slowing down the rate at which the virus will attack your immune cells."

And I tossed the pills into my throat, choking them down, praying that he was right.

For a week, I was too afraid to call or speak to anyone. I rolled my plan of attack around in my head like a nervous gambler fingering dice relentlessly, as if feeling them could signal the optimal moment for their release. Finally, I decided to first tell Antonio, and then Andrew.

I asked Antonio to meet me at a Cracker Barrel near my apartment. I wanted to go to a place that was big and loud and where we definitely wouldn't know anyone. And, there was something about the oversized rockers on the porch and the bright twists of candy in jars and fried apples and okra that made the place seem homey and safe. The kind of place that could, perhaps, with its cheerful folksiness, offset the fact that I was telling him that I was going to die and that he might die, too.

There is no kind of preamble to give news like this. So I didn't try. While Antonio and I waited for a table, sitting on the rocking chairs outside and looking across the parking lot, I told him plainly that I'd tested positive for HIV.

I had practiced telling him over and over in the same mirror in which I'd seen my face change forever. The one I'd broken in rage. But as the words flew out of my mouth like doves released from the inside of a wedding cake—supposedly light, airy and weightless, but in truth heavy, awkward and directionless—

it didn't go as planned. I had envisioned my face remaining peaceful and calm, the perfect balance between forgiveness and apology, as I still didn't know whether he'd given it to me, or if he even had it. Instead, it reflected the pain, anger and sorrow that pulled the muscles of my face awkwardly in opposing directions.

Neither of us said anything for a long time. We rocked self-consciously on the porch, the only sound the soft wooden squeak of the chairs. I remembered dreaming of being old one day and rocking away the end of my life. And now here I was at twenty-eight, doing just that.

I watched Antonio's face carefully as he absorbed the news. It didn't seem as if he knew. The fair skin on his brow wrinkled in genuine consternation beneath his tousled tuft of blond hair. The blue of his eyes deepened as welling tears (for himself? for me?) reddened the insides of his eyelids. In the days leading up to this moment, my mind had twisted and turned through all kinds of possibilities, including the idea that he had intentionally infected me in order to keep me by his side, just as a woman might try to force a man to stay with her by getting pregnant. I had ended our relationship abruptly and he had protested; I wasn't ready to date so soon after a divorce. It was hard to discern the true nature of his reaction through the shock that immobilized his face.

I asked Antonio, "Have you ever been tested for HIV?"

"No," he said tersely, but not necessarily defensively.

"Did you use IV drugs? Sleep with a man? With a prostitute? Were you really promiscuous?" I pressed him for the second time.

But even as the questions poured out of my mouth, I saw how ludicrous they were: I was HIV-positive and none of these things was true for me; none explained why I was now carrying the virus.

Before he had a chance to respond to my questions, the hostess came outside and said it would be a few more minutes before our table was ready. Wrapping her arms tightly around her body against the wind, she asked whether we were cold and if we wouldn't rather wait inside by the fire, where we could play checkers.

"Why not?" I said.

We sat by the fire, staring at the giant checkerboard. The oversized red and black discs and the simplicity of the moves of the game, which are intended to obliterate your opponent, seemed the perfect analogy for the idea of two people moving ever closer to the other's inner sanctum, tricking and deceiving and jumping over each other's lines of defense until one overtook the other. Was that what he had done to me?

Antonio struggled to regain his composure. As he did so, he thought out loud, trying to find an answer for how he could have gotten HIV. He asked me if I remembered the huge scar on his leg. I thought back to the first time I had noticed the jagged red line up his thigh. I had wondered about it, traced it with my finger, upset that he had suffered what must have been much pain. When I asked him about it, he had told me a story—a romantic fable of a contest of egos that involved drinking and riding rogue horses through the darkness of an Argentine night. While galloping across the pampas, he said, he fell and was impaled on a fence post. Hearing his cries, his friends placed him in the back of a truck and drove him to the nearest rural hospital, where, he said, he had been given blood.

"If I have it, and I gave it to you," he said, "I bet it's from that."

At the time, I thought it was almost gallant of him to entertain the notion—perhaps even assume—that it was more likely that he gave it to me than vice versa. The day would come when I would see this as evidence of his guilt.

I stared at his ice-blue eyes, remembering how I felt when I fell for him. We'd met at a polo game; we both played. One day, he invited me to help him exercise his horses. We were riding through a field and suddenly he was about twenty yards behind me, kneeling on the ground beside his horse. At first, I thought he'd fallen off. But he remounted and rode up beside me, handing me a wildflower he'd stopped to pick. I remember how as he held out his arm in the late afternoon sun, offering the bloom, the golden afternoon light illuminated the soft hair on his arm, which was sinewy with long muscles from a life spent working with horses. He seemed so sweet and healthy and strong. It was impossible to replace the images I had of him in my memory with the one in front of me now.

When we were finally seated at a table, we went through the motions of ordering and pretending to eat. We couldn't even talk about what it meant that I was HIV-positive. For one thing, I had no idea what it meant. For another, the weight of not knowing his status made all talk about HIV nearly impossible. So instead, we talked about anything else we could think of to fill the silence. I asked him inane questions. "How's your young mare coming along?"

"Good. I've already started playing her in practices."

"She looks like she's going to be a great one."

Our false cheer was too much to take. The waitress asked if we wanted dessert.

"Just the check," we both said quickly, and at once.

He smiled at me and I felt like throwing up. It would have been hard enough to see him so soon after I decided we didn't have a future together; under these circumstances, it was unbearable.

As we placed our napkins on the table and looked awkwardly around, my mind was a tangle of confusing thoughts. I hated him for maybe giving this to me. I hated having to tell him, thinking that maybe he was negative. I worried that if he had it, too, he'd want to get back together. What if he was the only person who'd be able to love me now?

He pulled on his coat, said he would get tested and let me know. We hugged good-bye. In my heart, I desperately wanted to hug him hard. But not knowing whether or not he'd given me the disease and whether he was repulsed by my HIV status stiffened my elbows. I kept space between us, as I once had kept space between myself and the boys I fox-trotted with in a church in Princeton so many innocent years ago.

The week that followed was a blur. I have tried many times to recall what I thought about while waiting for Antonio's result. I remember nothing except the mind-numbing worry that made it impossible to do anything except lie on my couch day after day and pray.

Each time I tried to take my HIV meds, I nearly choked to death. They stuck to each other, and then to the lining of my throat. I remembered that my doctor had given me the number of the Gay Men's Health Crisis, an AIDS service center in New York City. I dug the number out of my purse and decided to call them and see if this was typical.

The receptionist picked up.

"Hi. I'm not gay, and I'm not a man, but I just found out I have HIV and I . . . I really need some help," I stammered.

He assured me that the Gay Men's Health Crisis helped all people living with HIV. I told him that often I nearly vomited up any pills that I managed to get down my throat, which slammed shut as soon as it sensed the pills on my tongue. The man on the phone asked me if I believed in visualization. I said, "Kind of. But I'm not sure . . ."

He said, "Okay, first, take one pill at a time, so they don't stick together. Then, as you put each pill on your tongue, try to imagine it's a soldier you're sending in to fight a war inside your body."

Amazingly, it worked.

Each morning, midday and night, I would line up my little battalion of pills and talk to them. The big white ones were the legions of infantry I was sending into battle; the smaller one shaped like a diamond was the colonel. I was the general, giving them their marching orders. As I imagined their lethal power, suddenly my throat opened and they slid easily down my gullet. I no longer felt that they might come back up.

Antonio's test came back positive. He told me over the phone; I wasn't ready to see him again and was grateful that he called rather than come over. I could barely handle my own diagnosis; how was I going to help him with his? My mind went mad trying to evaluate how this had happened—to either of us. I thought about whether or not we should get back together; whether or not it made sense to be bound by the virus that threatened both our lives. There was a touch of Romeo and Juliet to our dark tale, but it seemed arbitrary and wrong to reconnect, or make a death pact, just because we were now maybe rendered off limits to all others.

When I tired of analyzing how, when, why this had all happened, and felt strong enough to set myself up for another body blow, I called Andrew. He'd moved to Connecticut after our divorce and though I felt that I should go see him in person, I honestly couldn't summon the strength. I needed to know that he was okay as soon as possible. He was incredibly calm when I shared the news and promised to call me as soon as he got the results of his test. I asked him if he wanted me to fly up and get the results with him. He said he would be okay.

It surprised me that both Antonio and Andrew were so calm when I told them. I wondered whether it was because they were in shock, sad for me, or frozen with worry about themselves. Probably all three.

Another week passed with agonizing slowness.

I worried that Andrew was positive, and that if he was, he'd never forgive me, nor would I forgive myself. I worried that if he was positive he'd tell everyone about it. And I was afraid that he'd given me the virus.

Finally, Andrew called and told me that he was HIV-negative and that he was coming to see me. He flew in, an act of great compassion, and made me laugh for the first time in weeks on the same couch on which I spent the whole first day after my diagnosis and on which I would later tell my mother that it looked like she was going to lose her daughter much sooner than she thought.

So it seemed that I had not passed on the virus to Antonio but that he'd given it to me. Given that Andrew and I had both tested negative before marrying—and that Antonio had HIV—much of the mystery had been solved. I didn't think Andrew had been unfaithful during our marriage—but I was doubly relieved when he tested negative: he was healthy and he hadn't cheated on me.

In a way, I felt better—I had been careful, and I had not, even inadvertently, hurt anyone. But freed of my fear that I would have another's blood on my hands, my mind turned to how, and perhaps why, Antonio had infected me, assuming he either knew his HIV status or had reason to believe that he could have been exposed to the virus.

I felt the first wave of anger toward Antonio. I did believe that he didn't know he was carrying HIV, but surely, he must have done something to get it—something he could have told me about that would have raised my defenses.

I spent uncounted days alone in my apartment, unable to

work, unable to think or feel or imagine or eat. It was the first of many times since my diagnosis that I would face the terrible demon of depression caused by feeling trapped in a body that was going to let me down by dying too young.

During those long days, I racked my brain for some clue about whether or not Antonio had known. I remembered a dinner we had at a Chinese restaurant. We were in an argument about whether or not I could match his level of emotional intimacy. He was Italian—all love and light and affection in public and I, according to him, was an ice princess.

Frustrated, he said in between bites of fried rice, "You don't know what love is. I would take a shot through my heart for you."

And he was right. I didn't know how to love like that—then. I wasn't ready to be loved by someone who would die for me. It seemed now I didn't have a choice in the matter.

After many nights of excruciating analysis of every moment we'd spent together, desperate to uncover a clue, I finally gave up. I was exhausted; I was sick and tired of trying to find the worst in someone I had loved. So I chose to believe Antonio—at least about his not knowing that he was carrying HIV. He must have known that something in his life had put him at risk, but again, all I had done was sleep with a nice guy who wasn't aware of his HIV status, so it was possible that all he did was sleep with a nice girl who wasn't aware that she was carrying the virus, either. It was possible that he was telling the truth.

CHAPTER
three

Finally, after three months of suffering alone, I couldn't take it anymore. I wanted desperately to tell my family but I didn't want to bring them pain. I tried repeatedly to tell my mom but every time I called to tell her, the same thing happened.

"Mom," I would say at some point in the conversation that seemed like a good moment to break the news that I had HIV. "I have something to tell you."

"Yes?" she would ask, with slightly more irritation each time I tried again.

"I . . . I . . . I bought a new horse," I'd said, the last time. "His name is Andiamo."

Somehow, despite the fact that I'm pretty sure she knew that something was terribly wrong, she could no more probe my unwillingness to come clean than I could share my truth with her.

She was right: I was slipping away. She had reason to worry— but not for any of the reasons she could have suspected. For once, the truth was much worse than even what a worried mother's imagination could conjure.

For three months after my diagnosis, I told myself that I could handle the disease myself. I really didn't want to burden my mom with either the fear she'd feel knowing I was positive, or her disappointment at learning I'd made such a critical mistake despite her incredible, careful mothering. But, week by week, my life came more unhinged. I wasn't working; I'd been trying to catch my breath after my divorce. The year before my diagnosis, I had left the local arts and entertainment magazine I helped found and was freelancing while planning my next career move. I was also training horses to help pay the bills. The news that I was dying didn't exactly make me want to send out my résumé. I'd feel guilty if someone hired me and I died a few months later. I needed the money—not to mention health insurance—but I was terrified that an employer would find out about my status and fire me.

It was really hard to care about the future when I didn't think I had one.

As those first months after my diagnosis rolled on, I withdrew from the world, never calling my friends back, turning down social invitations, feeling hopeless, helpless and alone. I apologized to my friends, connecting with them just enough to assure them that I was okay even though I wasn't. I made excuses to keep them from confronting me and making me tell them that there was indeed something wrong. When I ran into them in the grocery or tack store, I'd gather myself, paste on a huge smile and try to act as normal as I could. I felt like the manager of a bank that was being robbed by men in ski masks kneeling by my feet, holding guns to the small of my back.

Behind my stable veneer, I struggled to keep a grip on the simple realities of life—getting up, facing myself in the mirror, eating, taking my pills, going for a walk, taking more pills, eating, taking more pills, eating, bathing, breathing and trying to sleep.

While trying to hold on to a semblance of my sanity, I lost my hold on everything else.

When my mom told me that she was coming to visit me for the weekend, I knew that would be the right time to tell her.

She flew in a week later. My dad had similarly appeared the year before when he sensed that my marriage had fallen apart; I gave both my parents a lot of credit for being so perceptive and responsive. As for Tracy, because we are so close, I had to make up a story; there was no keeping my anguish from her. So when she repeatedly asked me, "What's wrong?" I said I was just stuck in a post-divorce depression, which was true.

After my mom arrived, I spent the whole weekend trying to pull off a charade of normalcy. We shopped—at flea markets, antique shops and T.J. Maxx. It was very early spring and, down south, the trees were beginning to leaf out. Over our first dinner, she questioned me about my future, quizzed me about my life plan. Considering that I'd gotten divorced not even a year after getting married, and her enormous year-long effort of planning the wedding and having to manage the social disaster of the marriage imploding so soon, she was incredibly understanding and patient with me. I knew I had deeply disappointed her, though she would never say so. That didn't make it any easier for me to tell her I had contracted HIV.

I tried to tell her so many times during the weekend. While we browsed through shops of old furniture, while making endless cups of tea in my kitchen and during car rides to the barn, the silence gnawed deeper into my gut. But though I willed the words to come out, they just wouldn't.

It wasn't until she was wheeling her suitcase toward the door of my apartment that desperation forced the truth out.

"Mom," I said. "I have something to tell you." I sat down on the small green love seat I had rescued from the curb. She took off her scarf and sat beside me. Who knew what she saw on my face, but if her own face reflected anything of mine, I looked scared to death.

"I don't know how to say this."

"What?" she demanded lightly. She summoned a little wave of anger to push her through the fear.

"I have HIV."

She said nothing, did nothing, for a minute or two. She stared into space, despondent as a wild animal that's been caught—and knows it will never get away. My heart throbbed in my chest; I could hear it swell and deflate ominously. Then a primal sound came from her mouth—the roaring wail of a mother lioness discovering her slain cub lying mutilated in the grass. It was an awful blend of wrenching agony and fear and emptiness and futility. A sound that said the things there are no words to describe. She paled as though blood was being wrung from her heart. I sat before her, feeling as if I was present at the discovery of my own dead body. She started breathing heavily. Her eyes were wide and dry. She didn't look at me for a while.

My heart felt as if it would stop.

I'm not dead yet, I wanted to say. I'm still here, alive and reasonably well. I touched her arm to prove my presence and she recoiled, not in fear or disgust, maybe just in disbelief that I was still breathing.

Then her face crumpled. And the tears came.

"What are we going to do?" she asked.

"We live. What else can we do before we die?" I said, trying to make myself believe my own words.

I grabbed her and held her and told her that I was going to be okay. Even though I wasn't. Or at least I didn't think I was, then. I rocked her back and forth on the couch, petting her head.

"I'm so sorry," I said. "I'm so, so sorry."

She raised her head once to look at me briefly as if to see if I was really still there.

Eventually, she inhaled enough air to force herself to sit up-right. She pushed her hair out of her eyes and avoided looking into mine.

"I'd better go," she said, standing shakily. "I don't want to miss my plane."

The reality that she wasn't going to stay and comfort me hit me like a Mack truck. I was so deeply ashamed.

"It wasn't drugs, Mom. It was a man. I didn't know. He didn't know," I said. "We're not bad people."

She stared at me and tried to carry her suitcase into the hall-way. But there was no strength in her arm and she left it for me as she walked to my car parked outside like someone who'd aged forty years in a minute.

We drove to the airport in silence. As we approached the ter-minal—the word stung me; everything pointed at death now—she took my hand.

"I need to go home and think about this. I need to talk to Frank about this. I'll call you," she said.

My stepfather was an oak of a man who would give her great solace. I nodded and bit my lip to keep from crying.

I got out of the car and took her luggage from the trunk. She hugged me hard and slumped into the airport.

One of my earliest memories of my mother was watching her ride a horse in Southern California, where we lived when I was seven. I was in a lesson, trotting in endless circles in the sandy arena on a roan mare, my legs barely long enough to bend and hang parallel to the horse's side. Gripping the horn of the saddle fiercely with fingers that were starting to blister, I saw a snowy white horse flying along the ridge above the riding ring. The rider was standing up in the saddle, balancing on the balls of her feet in the stirrups, freeing the horse to move effortlessly up the brush-covered hill.

The lesson stopped as we all watched my mother rein in her horse and guide him down the hill toward us. She approached us, electrically pretty, controlling her horse with gentle, nearly invisible movements of her legs and hands. The image of her like that was why I was torturing myself in my own sweat-stained saddle, trying to do as my instructor said: I wanted to be just like her.

To remember her then and to see her now was too painful. All the light and loveliness had left her and it was my fault.

I sat for a minute before driving away, checking to see if I felt better for having shared my secret. I did, but only because my pain had been transferred to another person. Now I had a new pain, one that came from knowing I had wounded someone I loved so much.

Looking in the rearview mirror, I saw a little rivulet of blood sliding down my lip where I'd bitten it, to keep from asking my mom to stay. I touched it with my finger and then—remembering that it was infected—rubbed it off with disgust onto a tissue.

I left the airport and slipped onto the highway, driving and driving and driving with nowhere really to go.

My mom had, as I expected, been bolstered by Frank, and she called me the next day, full of strength, cheer, resolution and reassurance. She insisted that I come home to New Jersey so she could help me with whatever it was I needed. We hadn't figured out much yet about how to cope with the disease, but it seemed right to be together while we tried to understand what to do next. So before I knew it, I was on a plane back to my hometown of Princeton, New Jersey.

When Tracy learned I was home, she came up from DC to see me. I wanted to tell her face to face, but I could see, as soon as she stepped off the train, that I wouldn't have to. My mother had already told her. Even when Tracy was still a small silhouette at the end of the very long platform, I could tell by the fierceness in her step that she'd already heard the news. She had come home to take care of me; to tell me it was going to be all right. She has always been stoic, calm—someone who just gets it done, no matter how hard, without a complaint. When she was close enough to see my eyes, she smiled. Standing before me, clutching the handle of her weekend bag tightly, she said simply, "We're going to kick this thing's ass."

I nodded firmly and gave her my bravest smile. I couldn't hug her or the tears would come and I wanted desperately to be big-sister strong.

Tracy said she was starving and asked if I wanted to get a Whopper. "Sure," I said.

We ordered as we always had—she rolled her eyes as I asked for extra pickles and no cheese on my cheeseburger. "What?" I shot back, "this is Burger King. They *want* me to have it my way."

When she laughed, I sensed for the first time the deep-rooted sadness that would stay with her from that day forward. She did an amazing job concealing her fear, but there was a streak of consternation in her that I doubted she'd ever shake.

We sat down and peeled the paper from our food. She spread the wrapper from her hamburger onto the brown plastic tray and

dumped both of our cartons of fries into the middle. Then, tearing up packets of Heinz 57, she made a little lake of ketchup
between us. We'd done this since I could remember. We talked
about anything but AIDS, and ate, and she casually dipped her
fries into my ketchup without any apparent concern for contracting my deadly disease. I loved her so much for not making me feel
like a leper.

"Have you told Dad?" she said, in the same flat practical tone
she might use to ask me if I'd filed my taxes.

"No. I don't know how."

She paused and ate her fries in precise, even bites.

"You're just going to have to tell him straight out. No 'Philadelphia shuffle,'" she said, referring to the phrase my dad used
as in, "Tell me what happened to the car. And I don't want
the Philadelphia shuffle." My dad liked the punch line first. He
liked to hear, for example, that you totaled the Oldsmobile station wagon and that no one was dead before getting into the
finer points of how you crashed the car because a wasp had
flown into your shoe. The whys, whens, hows and with whoms
always had to follow the whats when you were talking to my
dad, if you wanted his respect. And he always told us that he
would understand, and help, as long as we were up-front with
him about any problem.

My dad was also my friend and, through his divorce from my
mother, he and I had resolved most of the issues that stood between us when I was a teenager and in my early twenties. I had
enormous admiration for his work ethic and moral compass and
I had tried all my life to meet the standards he set for me.

Once, when I got nearly all A's on a report card, he called me
into his library. He placed my report card on his desk and staring
at it asked, "What happened?"

Dumbstruck, I said, "What do you mean?"

He laid his fingertip on the sole B+ and said, "What happened here?"

I wanted to say that it had been kind of a tricky year, I hated the teacher and I had fallen hopelessly in love with the guy who sat next to me in class and the combination wasn't conducive to optimizing my attention span or my ability to absorb the finer points of advanced placement physics. But excuses weren't allowed.

"I don't understand," I said instead. "Why do I have to have straight A's? A B+ is a good grade."

"It is, for some people," he said. "If I thought you were only capable of getting straight C's and you tried your hardest and got straight C's, I would be proud of you. But you can get straight A's and you didn't."

I had no idea how to tell a man who believed me capable of the highest standards in every aspect of my life that I had faltered and made a mistake that was going to cost us all a lot of money, social disgrace, agony and probably my life.

I had called my father to tell him I was coming home for a visit and that I'd like to come over to talk to him about something. He still lived in the sprawling stone farmhouse just outside of Princeton where I had grown up. As I drove down our pine-tree-lined driveway past the kennel, the barn and the entrance to the woods where I'd spent countless hours walking the dogs or cooling my feet in the stream on hot summer days while doing my homework, it seemed unfathomable to me that all those blissfully happy days of my youth and early adulthood could have led me to the point of having to make the confession I was about to share with my dad. I met his eyes through the glass panes of the door. He'd heard my car and had come to let me in. We went into the sunroom, where our family had had lunches together on weekends.

As Tracy and I agreed, I told him straight out that I had something difficult to tell him. I suggested he sit down, which he did, on a wicker chair, gripping its sides as he waited to hear what I had to say.

Now it was my turn to brace myself. I also sat down and, before I chickened out and ran out the door, said quickly, "Something bad has happened, Dad. I got tested and found out I have HIV."

As soon as I'd said the words, I dropped my gaze to the floor. When I looked up again, he had let go of the chair and folded his arms against his chest. An Annapolis grad and a captain in the Marine Corps—a man who had slept with his head uphill in the muddy jungles of Vietnam so water wouldn't run into his nostrils who spent summers on destroyers and submarines and leading a combat platoon of young men through Borneo on training exercises—he took the news as a man trained for war might. His ruddy, leading-man face with twinkling blue-gray eyes, thick, imposing brows and a square jaw barely registered the pain he surely felt. His jaw stayed rigid and his eyes remained fixed on a point over my shoulder. In mere seconds, he moved from despair to battle plan.

"You will survive this," he said quickly with a conviction that surprised me. "I will get you the best medical care possible. You don't have to worry about a thing."

Except maybe dying a slow, excruciating and humiliating death, I thought, but did not say. I had spent the bulk of my life trying to please my dad. Not in a crazy, obsessive way. I simply admired him and knew that if I could achieve his stamp of approval, I would have achieved a great thing. I couldn't even tell him I was sorry. Because there were no words to express just how sorry I was for not turning out the way both of us had hoped I would.

I sat down in the chair facing him and thought back on the many happy days my family had had in that sunroom after doing our Saturday chores around the farm. I could practically still hear my mom calling to my dad from the kitchen, asking whether or not he wanted pickles with his hoagie, and my sister's exasperated, elongated "But, whhhhhhyyyyyy????" when my mom told us we had to trim the forsythia or pull the dead stalks from the beds of day lilies.

I finally looked at my dad's face and we stared at each other while I nodded, trying not to cry, trying to show resolve. He squinted ever so slightly, and I thought I could just make out the pain that was beginning to surface in his face. But I could also see that his respect and concern for me were trumping his anguish. There was also still love in his eyes—and I promised myself silently I would do everything I could to maintain my health for as long as I could, and be as little of a burden as I could, emotionally and financially, to him and everyone else in my family as payback for their amazing support.

I wanted to sit in the sunny room and soak up his strength all day. But I knew I needed to leave so he could break down.

He hugged me good-bye. He patted my back and his affection came out as several brusque slaps on my shoulder blades. I appreciated the firmness of his touch. Softness had never worked well for either of us.

CHAPTER
four

After visiting my family in Princeton, it quickly became clear to me that I wasn't going to be able to stay in Atlanta and deal with HIV by myself. After things fell apart with Andrew, there wasn't much reason to stay, anyway; as a new divorcee my social life had all but dried up and it seemed necessary to put some distance between myself and Antonio. Though in my heart of hearts, I was sure he hadn't intentionally infected me, nothing could take away the fact that I was probably going to die.

So I decided to move back to New Jersey—and in with my mom and Frank. The months of silent agony seemed like distant memories once I'd told my family and received their support. It didn't take long after disclosing to them to realize that I'd needed more than just knowing that they knew I was living with HIV—I needed to be near the people who would help me through the unthinkable process of battling my end.

I told my few friends that I was leaving, claiming that I needed to regroup post-divorce. I think, in a way, they were relieved not to feel the pressure of including me as a fifth, seventh or ninth wheel in the nearly exclusively happily-married-coupledom that they all lived in.

I packed up my apartment and made arrangements for my horses to be shipped professionally to Princeton in an eighteen-wheeler. The truck had an air ride and the driver would stop halfway to New Jersey and spend the night on a farm where the horses could stretch their legs.

I've ridden horses since I was six years old and all my life a mere whiff of a stable or a sweaty horse has calmed my nerves like a handful of Valium. Now, more than ever, I needed that horsepower.

When moving day came, I wrapped the horses' legs in protective shipping boots, loaded them in the trailer and filled their water buckets with familiar water. And I told Bob, the driver, that I'd meet him, three days later, in New Jersey.

With my own possessions packed tightly into a U-Haul, I trundled slowly northward, glad to be headed home. Listening to the radio, just outside of Atlanta, I heard, with horror, that there was a huge storm coming; they were calling for three feet of snow. Living so far south of the Mason-Dixon Line, I forgot that there could still be extreme weather where I was headed, and I hadn't thought to check. I called Bob and asked what we should do.

"How are your winter driving skills?" he said with a laugh.

I'd been in the truck just half an hour and my arms were already exhausted from turning the big awkward wheel, trying desperately not to veer into other lanes of traffic.

"Well, to be honest, I'm not that good at driving a big truck," I said. I had some experience driving horse trailers and polo rigs but nothing like what I was in now—and certainly not in the snow.

"Well, you just take your time and I'll get your horses there safely and we'll see you when we do," he said.

That sounded fine to me, but some dear family friends had graciously offered to house my horses in their barn on the farm next to ours for the remainder of the winter, and I really needed to be there to ensure that the horses got settled in smoothly. My mother, who planned to meet me at the barn to help unload the horses, had made me promise not to be late. Rightfully so, as she wasn't confident that she could handle thousands of pounds of horseflesh that had been locked up in a truck for three days on her own. Nor should she have been.

The snow started not long after I crossed over the state line into North Carolina. At first, it was a gentle sifting of doily-like flakes; then, more like a pillow fight when the down's burst out of its sacking. By the time I reached Virginia, it was a blinding white crosshatching that slowed the light traffic to a crawl.

I called my mom.

"Hi, Mom," I said, trying to have an upward lilt in my voice.

"Hello," she said seriously. "Have you seen the weather?"

"Well, actually, I'm in it," I said.

"I think you're going to have to stop at your aunt's house in Lynchburg," she said.

Normally, I would have been excited to visit my mom's sister. But the thought of facing family members made me nervous. I knew I'd have to act excited and pretend that things were great, and tell them that I was simply moving home to recover from the divorce. I was nervous that they'd see right through me. And I didn't want my mom to have to handle the horse drop-off alone.

"Okay," I said reluctantly. "I'll call Aunt Kay and we'll stay in touch."

"Drive carefully, please," she said. "I love you."

I called my Aunt Kay, my mother's sister, and my Uncle John, who were thrilled to hear that I would be visiting. Many long hours of white-knuckled driving later, I arrived at their house. They lived in a large white antebellum-esque mansion with columns framing their massive entryway; their house was impeccably decorated. After taking my bags upstairs to the guest room, I joined them in the kitchen. Kay had all sorts of foods simmering in pots on the stove, and she had already set the table with the family silver. I felt so guilty that they'd prepared such a celebratory spread on such a dire occasion.

My Aunt Kay is an effusive southern woman with the energy and joie de vivre of an entire sorority. You could be about to commit suicide and then encounter my aunt, and within seconds, forget your troubles entirely. But even though her take on life was just what I needed, I couldn't imagine polluting their world—a world of debutante balls and long afternoons by the pool—with something as grotesque as HIV. Then I remembered that they didn't know. And it was nice to experience one final illusion of my life—that I was totally okay—before I went home to face my new grim reality.

We sat around their table and devoured the comfort food Aunt Kay had cooked for us. We ate until we were stuffed and drank bottles of white wine. They asked me all about my move back to Princeton, and when I told them how much I missed the East Coast they laughed and went on about how they could never live anywhere else but the South. Yes, with a capital S. We talked about how their golden retriever, Buffy, had developed a habit of carrying bricks around in her mouth (which explained her missing front teeth). We talked about Tracy's impending graduation from law school, and my cousins John, Christopher and Meagan. During dessert, Uncle John, an oncologist, regaled us with tales from med school. He told stories from the days of his OB/GYN rotation.

The details of the stories are now blurred (you'll see why in a moment) but I think one involved him standing beside the doctor as a baby shot out of a young mother—into his unsuspecting arms.

Suddenly, the notion that I'd never be able to have a baby hit me like a ton of Buffy's bricks. I tried to summon levity and laugh with Kay and John, who were howling at his punch line. I tried focusing on their grinning faces as a wave of nausea came over me. For the first time since the day of my diagnosis, the news that I was never going to have a child washed over me like a deluge.

I don't remember passing out. When I came to, I was lying on the couch with a cool washcloth on my head, Aunt Kay's soft hands around my now shoeless feet and, Uncle John's strong hand on my shoulder.

They looked concerned—and relieved.

"Thank heavens you're okay!" my aunt exclaimed in her southern twang.

If only they knew.

I slept deeply and in the morning, armed with some aspirin and Diet Coke, set out trying to beat the horses to New Jersey.

The snow had rendered the countryside idyllic, if treacherous.

Somewhere in Virginia, while rolling up and down the gently undulating hills, I noticed that people were playing in the snow. In the vacuum I'd lived in since finding out about the HIV, I'd forgotten that other people still experienced joy and frivolity and joked and dreamed and felt carefree.

I was watching a string of kids pull each other gleefully through the snow on Flexible Flyers when I first spied the horse. It was white and standing in the middle of the snowy road, looking confused. I slammed on the brakes, causing the truck to slide sideways. Thankfully, the drifts left by an earlier plow provided a buffer and I ground the U-Haul to a halt without crashing. I thought about how ironic it would have been to kill this horse because I was driving too fast, trying to save my own horses.

I stepped out of the car and walked up to the horse, who stood quietly looking at me through thick black lashes. It exhaled as I approached, like a dragon, offering fair warning.

I extended my hand and slowly reached for his head. I was worried that he'd gallop off across the highway, into the lanes of oncoming traffic. Not that many other people were crazy enough to be driving in the blizzard. Why, I wondered, did strange creatures in need always appear in front of me whenever I was in a rush? Was the universe trying to protect me, using my rescue instinct as a means to keep me from needing to be rescued myself?

He didn't move as I sidled up to him and pulled off my belt, slowly so as not to spook him, and buckled it around his head. I led him off the highway with my makeshift halter, and called the police.

He nuzzled me and I wondered whether someone was missing him.

The cops arrived minutes later—but the spinning red and blue lights of the squad car frightened the horse; he reared and escaped my grip. I ran off after him in the snow. He didn't go far and I was able to catch him again. I trudged through the drifts, horse in tow, back to the policemen.

One of the officers stepped up.

"What would you like us to do?" he said.

"Find out where he lives and take him there," I said.

"Where was he, when you found him?" the other cop asked.

"Right there," I said, pointing to the middle of the highway. "He came from that direction." I pointed at his hoof prints, which had come from across the highway.

"Good thing you got him out of the road," the other said.

"Yeah," I said. "I almost crashed trying not to run him over."

"Here," I motioned to the first policeman. "Please take him from me. I'm late."

"I don't know anything about horses," he said, stepping back.

"He's very gentle. He'll follow you wherever you take him," I said.

The officer gingerly took hold of my belt fastened around the horse's face and, when the horse stayed calm, smiled, pleased that he could control the beast beside him. The horse pushed his head against the officer's leg and he nearly fell down in the snow. He giggled and said, "Ah, come on now, boy!" It never ceases to amaze me how the willing obedience and trust of an animal as large and powerful as a horse can make people childlike again.

I thanked the cops and wished them luck and continued on my way.

As I drove off, I wondered if the horse was a metaphor for my inability to see what was right in front of me. For the next two hours, my mind wandered back through all the time I'd spent with Antonio, trying to pinpoint whether I had refused to see the obvious: that Antonio was lying or already sick from HIV, or both. Had I been too blinded by love to notice? I remembered re-peatedly noticing a sore on his leg that took a long time to heal. I recalled thinking it was strange and even asked him about it. He said it was from his polo boots and that it wouldn't heal because he wore them every day.

I also remembered one of the many summer evenings we spent at our polo barn together. I'd kept my horses with his. I'd been looking for a syringe to give my horse a shot of penicillin, and been unable to find it. I kept tons of them in a plastic zip-pered bag in my tack trunk, and suddenly, they were all gone. He said he'd used them for one of his horses, but something in his tone didn't sit well with me. But I never imagined that there'd be any reason to be suspicious of him. Now, with the perspective of hindsight, I wondered whether he could have used those needles for himself. Was that the white horse in the snow?

By the time I finally got to Princeton, my horses had already arrived and my mom had unloaded them without my help. Our neighbor's driveway was nearly a half-mile long, which meant my mom had walked miles in knee-high snow and whipping wind while holding on to rearing, frightened and confused horses.

Later, my mom told me that Milagro, my young paint mare, refused to step down the ramp into the strange whiteness on the ground and that it had taken encouragement with a cattle prod to get her moving. Hitting the cold snow, she'd bounced like a caribou on crack down the driveway, while my mom tried desperately not to let go.

I parked the U-Haul and stepped out into the snow. When I entered the barn, I found my mom sweeping the floors, pressing the broom down so hard that she sent stray pieces of hay and grain flying with each stroke. She had managed to get all my horses into their stalls and to feed them. Knowing what a hassle it all must have been for her, I felt a pang of guilt rise in my stomach, and at the same time, a strange sense of relief to have an artificial reason for the tension we felt at the first awkward homecoming. Before, it was always a celebration to come home—it was someone's birthday, a holiday, a vacation. To come home to die? That was no cause for joy.

My mom looked at me, exhausted, and propped the broom against the wall. "I'm going home to take a hot shower and to get some sleep," she said. "Your room's all ready for you. We'll talk in the morning, okay? Glad you made it home safely." She gave me a hug and a kiss. And with that she was gone.

I went into Andiamo's stall and sat down on an overturned water bucket by his front feet. He lowered his chocolate brown muzzle to my face and shoved me gently. He exhaled on my head

and pric ked me with his whiskers. I talked softly to him, fee
calmer and calmer with every one of his molasses-ridden bre
my face.

Back in Atlanta, when I struggled to stay out of th
hole of depression dug by the inescapability of my disea
fear of a slow, painful, embarrassing demise, Andiam
me. No matter how down I got, I still had t
him, clean his stall and take him out to th
me something to live for, by forcing m
the house and into the healing rays
darkness at bay.

stand at the gat
d his head

...diamo instantly. I told the groom I'd take him bu... ...he said

...I have to ask the owner of the polo team if he was ...uly f...

...ear after seeing him in Florida, I learned he'd been sold ...on the farm of a local horse trainer in Georgia. I called ...er whether she still had the horse; she did and said I ...ome and see him.

...arm on a cool rainy day. The trainer won-

...for, since several other riders had said

...orthless.

...indow and saw a bunch of rain-

...he far side of the pa...

...e wire

*   *   *

Sitting on top of Andiamo changes the way I see the world. I have been climbing onto the backs of horses since I was six years old; I have almost never found a better replacement for the feeling of empowerment that comes when I sling my right foot over a horse's back and settle gently into the saddle.

Through all the years that Andiamo and I have risked our lives together jumping at twenty miles an hour over fences made out of stacks of river rocks, fallen trees or railroad ties, I have never not trusted him for a second. As we gallop to the base of a hulking jump, if I feel that we might not have the right approach or I can't see the take-off spot, I close my eyes and let him feel his way up and over the obstacle. Though it is counterintuitive to let go when things seem to be out of control, it is sometimes exactly what one needs to do. If I grabbed the reins and tried to force the situation, we would probably crash. So I left it to him, and the universe, to carry us safely to the other side.

This was one of countless lessons he unknowingly imparted to me. When I bought him, I thought he came into my life to take me to the upper levels of Three-Day Eventing—a sport that's like an equestrian triathlon. But he came, instead, to teach me about things more important than the pursuit of a blue ribbon—things like humility and how to overcome doubt, pain and mind-numbing fear.

In the stall next door, Milagro, my other horse, pawed; she could hear my voice and was looking for treats. She was all white except for a cherry-brown cap over the crown of her head and ears, a shield on her chest and one on each flank, just over the area where the back legs met her body; it was a rare pattern of markings that Native Americans called a Medicine Hat paint. The legend about Medicine Hat paints says that no one who rides one can be killed. The myth was perpetuated largely because chiefs often rode the horses with these flashy markings and the chiefs rarely got close enough to the front lines of battle to be killed. Little did I know when I bought her that I'd have need for her magical life-sustaining qualities, too.

Listening to her bump around her stall looking for me and feeling Andiamo's hot breath, I allowed my tears to fall freely. I had vowed to try to control my weak moments in front of my family, especially now that I was going to be living with my mom and Frank. I didn't want to upset them any more than I already had. I had to be strong. But in the barn, with my horses, I let myself go, crying as I had never cried before and feeling the warm, reassuring comfort of their steady breath and unflinching stillness.

CHAPTER
five

My mom and Frank had only been married two years when I moved in with them and I didn't know Frank very well. I can't imagine what it would be like to hear that your spouse's twenty-eight-year-old, HIV-positive child is coming home to live with you. But if it upset Frank, he never showed it.

As I moved into the house, carrying box after box into the spare bedroom my mother had made up for me—a near exact replica of my childhood room—Frank cheerfully bantered with me about the drive, the horses and the weather.

My mom and Frank had built a large French country home on a piece of land that Frank had inherited. It already had a full garden of mature specimen trees and glorious five-foot-high rhododendron bushes. My bedroom looked out on a circle of grass inside the looped driveway; through the tree line at the far edge of the property, I could just make out the black-and-white shapes of a large herd of dairy cows grazing in the field.

Even though Frank and my mom never seemed hesitant about living with me, I worried constantly. I worried I would give them

HIV, that they were secretly worried I would give them HIV, that they didn't want their friends to know I had it, that their friends would find out I had it. The list was endless. I scrubbed my dishes until the paint nearly chipped in water that seared the skin of my hands. I used about a half gallon of bleach in every load of my laundry—determined to kill the virus.

At first, I wondered whether I could give them AIDS by double dipping my Tostitos in the salsa or running my knife over the same brick of butter. Although my doctors had assured and reassured me that HIV is not passed through casual contact, I was petrified that we would be the example that proved everyone wrong. Though there was overwhelming proof that HIV could not jump between people during a hug, in the spin cycle of the wash or on a brick of soap, it took living that reality to believe it. And how would I know, anyway? It wasn't like my mom and Frank were going to repeatedly get tested for HIV.

It had been eleven years since Ryan White was banned from school for having HIV, five years since Magic Johnson's famous public disclosure in 1991, and two years since Pedro Zamora shockingly announced that he was HIV-positive to his co-stars on *The Real World*; but the stigma surrounding the disease was still overwhelming. Those were still the days when—though people might have evolved to being able to talk about Tom Hanks's role as an HIV-positive lawyer in *Philadelphia* at the dinner table—no one thought that AIDS would actually happen to anyone *at* the dinner table. Having HIV meant to many people that you were gay, a junkie or a whore. Even Magic, who everyone loved, was after all an NBA star—the implication being that he'd slept with many women. People made an automatic link between HIV and promiscuity, even though that wasn't necessarily true.

My mom and Frank never flinched or showed any concern that HIV was whirling around their house, or lurking dangerously on the countertops. I still remember the first time Frank, who was eating liver one night during the first week I was home, on discovering I'd never tried the organ meat, slid his plate down the table until it was in front of me and said, "Go on, take a bite." I didn't, but not because of HIV. It was because the idea of eating an organ designed to rid the body of toxins repulsed me.

As we read magazines together in the late afternoons with our tea, my mom sat on the couch nestled right up beside me; she kissed me on the face when I was sad and hugged all my sheets and clothes to her chest when taking them to the basement to wash them. And on the few occasions when I couldn't keep my pain to just the horses, she'd wipe the tears off my face with her bare hand, grab me in her arms and say, "Come on now, you're going to be fine."

The first time Frank spoke harshly to me, I was relieved. Over breakfast on a Sunday morning, he curtly asked whether I'd mind taking off my cowboy boots before traipsing down the wood-floored hallway that ran directly over his bedroom in the middle of the night. It must have seemed weird to him when I beamed a big smile back at him. It was just that since I felt so different after finding out I had HIV, I desperately wanted to be treated like anyone else.

I knew how lucky I was to be accepted by my dad, my sister, my mom and Frank. Just after I was diagnosed, and before I told my family, thanks to the help of the doctor who diagnosed me, I'd connected with a support group of gay, HIV-positive men in Atlanta. My doctor suggested that I attend their group because, at the time, there were no HIV/AIDS support groups for straight women. We met in the living room of one of the men's homes. During my first meeting, we talked about going home to see our families for the holidays and what that could mean for those of us whose families knew our HIV status—and those whose families did not. We all feared being ostracized, pitied, feared, and judged. To everyone around me, I seemed healthy, affluent, well educated, privileged. I'd gone to private school. I had a degree from Trinity College in Hartford, Connecticut, and, post-graduation, had run with a fast, wealthy and international crowd in New York City, where I lived until Andrew and I got married. I'd worked at CBS News and at several top advertising agencies. I had all the makings of a highly successful young woman. Which made it particularly hard to admit that I had derailed my chances of success by getting a terminal disease.

That first day, I walked stiffly into the circle of southern gay men who eyed me from head to toe. As I looked around the room, I wondered: Could I really relate to these men? What could we possibly have in common? As it turned out, nearly everything.

We all worried about rejection, protecting our partners, and whether or not we'd ever experience sexual pleasure again. We worried that people we wanted to date would find out, by accident, that we had HIV before we had a chance to tell them, or that after we did, our disease would be a turnoff and they'd run away. And we all lamented that even if a partner was willing to be with us sexually despite the HIV, AIDS was anything but an aphrodisiac; we would struggle to banish thoughts of HIV from our own heads if we ever hoped to regain the fullness of our sex lives.

I felt really awkward at first. I had never been to a support group of any kind, and had very limited experience pouring my heart out to people I barely knew. And I wasn't very comfortable talking about my body or sex life, especially to a group of men. As man after man shared the most intimate fears and confessions, I sat absolutely still and expressionless with my hands folded primly and anxiously on my crossed legs. But finally, during one man's story, I came undone.

He shared what happened the first time he went home to Baton Rouge for Thanksgiving after being diagnosed with AIDS. He'd told his well-to-do and well-educated parents that he was living with HIV; they were supportive and loving. He described how he had cried with relief as they embraced him—literally and figuratively. He left, full of joy. When he was about half an hour away, he realized he'd forgotten his overnight bag. When he got back to his parents' house, he found his mom burning his sheets in an oil drum in the backyard. Peering into the fire, he saw that she'd also thrown away the silver cutlery from which he'd eaten his Thanksgiving dinner.

His mother was devastated that he'd found her cooking his sheets. Through her tears, she tried to explain that she thought that was the only way to keep her house—and the rest of the family— HIV free. As he talked, I watched the man's chin fall slowly from the high defiant jut where it was when he started telling the story until it was tucked sadly down on his chest like a bird that's put its head under its wing. And I just lost it. This proud, strong man had tried so hard to understand and forgive his mother, but who could withstand watching your mom set fire to your bedclothes? I unfolded my hands and legs and walked across our little circle of chairs and sat by his feet, hugging his legs. One by one, the other men joined me until we embraced in a single ball of communal grief, crying both for his pain, and for the pain it caused in us, fearing what might lie in store for us at our own families' houses.

I had to get my blood checked every three months to see if, and how well, the drugs were suppressing the virus, and it was at a hospital, of all places, that I experienced my first bout of HIV-related fear and stigma.

Everything was fine, at first. The nurse who was supposed to draw my blood swabbed the inside of my arm, tied the rubber tubing around my bicep, then turned to my chart to check what vials she needed to fill. Seeing what she was testing me for, she stopped putting on her gloves and said fiercely, "I'm not going to draw *your* blood. You have HIV." She left the room in a bustle of starched white uniform and I sat there, dumbfounded and immobilized until my arm started going numb. Finally, realizing no one was coming back, I pulled the rubber tubing off my arm, stood up, put on my coat and walked out to reception. The receptionist was on the phone and didn't even look up as I walked slowly out of the office. I felt like a bird that had flown into a window. Stunned and sore, hurt by something I never saw coming.

Going down in the elevator I felt sick to my stomach and afraid. How the hell was I supposed to survive if even the medical community refused to help me?

Luckily, the man in my support group had taught me that in order to recover from that kind of incident I'd first need to realize that I didn't deserve to be treated like that. After recovering from the shock of the backyard bonfire, he said, he printed out a ton of material about the facts surrounding HIV transmission and mailed it to his mother with a letter asking her to go to his doctor with him, which she eventually did. The next time he went home, she didn't burn anything.

I finally got the nerve to admit to my doctor what had happened when he called and asked why he never got my blood work results; in turn, he contacted the hospital, reported the nurse and found me a great one who not only drew my blood but made me feel like just another patient while doing it.

But I wondered: What happens to HIV-positive people who can't find the right kind of support? Do they ever speak to their families again? Do they ever go back to the doctor?

I think because she felt powerless to save her dying child, my mother tried to hyper-control other aspects of her life. And sometimes, mine. She patiently corrected my grammar, made suggestions about my diet (I should eat more pasta! and butter!), and questioned whether or not riding horses was a smart thing to do given The Situation.

But if living with my mom at the age of twenty-eight was sometimes stressful, it was also a godsend. I spent long nights armed with white wine, sitting on the terrace with my mom and Frank, watching the sun set behind their magnificent garden. As birds zipped from feeder to feeder, we talked politics, pop culture and gardening; none of us imagined that one day, years later, they'd throw a wedding party for my second marriage, on that same terrace. That first year, none of us ever dared speak of the future.

It was strange never to refer to things to come. But it was also relaxing, in a way, not having to plan for a lifetime of tomorrows. Embracing the notion of an early death meant that I was exempt from all kinds of nastiness associated with old age. It simplified my concerns. I had no need to siphon my paychecks into a 401(k), would not get wrinkles or end up alone, in adult diapers, trying to remember who I was one day.

If you'd asked me before I contracted HIV what I would have done with myself if someone had told me I was going to die prematurely, I'm sure I would have concocted all kinds of wild endings to my life. Become a professional kite surfer in Mauritius! Pursue enlightenment in the Himalayas! Ride a yak! My imagined end-of-life scenarios changed settings frequently (Morocco, Costa Rica, the Galapagos) but most of them involved me wearing little clothing, never washing my hair, eating birthday cake three times a day, never returning a phone call from anyone with whom I didn't want to speak and maintaining no agenda so I could wander from moment to moment through the day.

The reality was different, though, in part because when you are told that your days are numbered, you understand, for the first time perhaps, how amazing your everyday life already is. Suddenly, you don't need to jet to sapphire seas; after my diagnosis, my favorite stretch of woods was every bit as magical as a footprint-free stretch of sugar-fine sand on a faraway atoll.

It's hard to radically change your life just because you have an awareness of how, and when, it might end. The thought of my imminent demise sucked all the buoyancy and adventure from my spirit; I just wanted to rest and spend quality time with my family. Also, I was afraid to do anything too physically challenging, lest I accelerate the coming of the end.

I often thought about what I would say on my deathbed. I tried over and over to write the words I'd say to my family while I lay dying, but I could never get past the first sentence. And while it made sense to say now what I might not be able to when the time I had to say my final good-byes finally came, there was never a non-crisis moment that seemed right for my farewells.

So, instead, I just mostly pretended it wasn't happening.

I combated the fear of my death by being determined to live as fully as I could, while I had life. I indulged slightly more than I normally would in things I formerly found frivolous. Taking handfuls of pills each day and worrying each morning that that day would begin my official demise, I allowed myself more indulgences than I did before I was diagnosed. If I wanted butterscotch for breakfast, I had it.

To avoid thinking of dying, I sometimes occupied myself with inane things like what on earth I was going to wear to the Museum of Natural History's winter dinner dance. An old friend from my New York days had heard I was back in the area and invited me to go with him.

I found a dress for the ball in a vintage store. I have always loved secondhand things. I think it has to do with my own feelings, and fears, about myself being less than perfect—and being discarded. There is so much wonderful furniture and stunning clothing and accessories, not to mention animals and children, in the world that people have decided have no value. It gives me great pleasure rescuing these unwanted things. Not only do I get to bring beautiful, valuable objects into my world at little expense, but doing so offers the satisfaction of giving something a second chance at life. The otherwise unwanted living creatures I find offer a unique appreciation for being taken in. But even the inanimate objects seem glad to be saved.

Not all old things make a successful transition to the modern world. The dress I bought for the winter dance was a strapless, aqua chiffon gown with gathered fabric that came to peaks above my breasts, pointing at my throat. Its skirt was full and dragged behind me on the floor. It was either vaguely Dior-esque circa the 1970s or a total fashion tragedy. I really couldn't tell which. It had been so long since I'd gotten really dressed up—the last time I could remember doing so was for my wedding. And skinny as I was, I didn't really have the '40s Hollywood body it was designed for.

Because HIV had done such a whammy on both my self-esteem and confidence I could hardly see myself clearly. So I swished into the sunroom one Sunday morning where Frank was reading the paper and asked him what he thought of my new old dress.

He burst out laughing.

My face fell and my arms hung limp by my sides. Sensing my distress, he said, "You are a very beautiful woman. But that dress doesn't flatter you at all." And then he chuckled some more.

Before I knew it I was laughing, too. In that moment of pure honesty, part of me wanted to ask him what he *really* thought about my having contracted HIV. But as desperate as I was to know the unedited truth, I didn't have the courage to ask him. Just like my mortality, there were some things I wasn't ready to face fully yet.

CHAPTER
six

While I was trying to maintain the appearance that all was well in my life, my family and I had to address the reality of my illness behind closed doors.

Since returning home, I'd spent a lot of time up late at night on the Internet reading about HIV. At first, I read about the virus in small doses, trying not to be terrified by notions like oral thrush, wasting syndrome or Kaposi's sarcoma (cancerous lesions that appear as dark spots on the body, mercifully something women got less frequently than men). I had loved studying science at school and tried to digest, through the lens of my scientific curiosity, the descriptions of how HIV docks onto receptors of the CD4 cell, enters the cell and, through a process called reverse transcriptase, basically steals the host cell's DNA, thus enabling the birth of a new viral particle. By doing so, it kills the cells of your immune system. Your body works frantically to replace them, but HIV uses them to replicate faster than the body can manufacture enough healthy cells to keep HIV in check. Eventually, HIV takes over and your immune system can no longer produce enough CD4 cells to stay on top of the virus and is weakened to a critical point.

I learned that HIV stands for human immunodeficiency virus. And that it is the name for the retrovirus that causes AIDS, which stands for acquired immunodeficiency syndrome. AIDS refers to the state of your body after HIV has wiped out your immune system. So you can be HIV-positive, or living with HIV, but not yet have AIDS.

It was frightening not only to read about what could, and likely would, happen to me before I died, but also to realize how little was known then about the disease, and how powerful the virus was.

Desperately hungry for information, I went to Borders bookstore and perused the health section for books about AIDS. I carried a stack of them to the checkout counter and, laying them on the counter, whispered to the cashier, "I'm doing a research project on AIDS." The irony was, she hadn't been looking at me like I could have AIDS. I was anything but the typical poster child for the virus.

I kept the books in a vintage suitcase in my bedroom. Not that anyone was visiting me at my mom's house; I tried not to highlight the fact I was living with my mom and step-dad though I was nearly thirty.

My mom read the books, too, and Frank always clipped articles about AIDS from the newspaper for me. My dad and Tracy also did research. But everything we read painted the same grim picture. The end appeared to be coming no matter what and it wasn't going to be pretty.

But for all my inevitable thoughts about death, somehow, even in those early days of living with HIV, part of me was convinced that HIV wasn't actually going to kill me. And while I had been far from a model of perfect health (despite a lifetime of sports—riding, tennis, field hockey, rowing crew and rugby—my breakfasts often consisted of Twizzlers and Diet Coke), I inherently believed in my constitutional fortitude. I continued to get my blood count tested and my mom worked furiously to find me the best doctor in the country who had access to the most cutting-edge treatments. But as extra insurance, I decided to pursue some alternative healing. I had gone to an acupuncturist for a pain in my neck once and the treatment had helped immensely. While the idea of paying someone to stick needles in me seemed absurd and painful, I was willing to try anything to stay well.

I went to the offices of Bert Rinkel in New Hope, Pennsylvania. His healing workshop is situated along the Delaware River, which separates Pennsylvania and New Jersey. Bert had a large white beard and a thick crown of white hair. His voice was soothing and low.

He invited me into a room full of crystals and mysterious ancient Chinese charts, bells, abalone shells, a wooden eagle, gongs, drums and a jar of something he called "moxa"—dried mugwort that he balled up, set on the ends of the needles and set on fire.

He couldn't cure my HIV, he said, but he could help me fight it by bolstering my immune system and detoxifying my body to cleanse it of the residual toxins from the medicines I took to fight HIV.

In our intake meeting, he asked me a lot of questions about my physical history—as well as questions about the state of my mind. I could sum it up in a single word: delicate.

I wanted to tell him that some days, the blue of the sky blinded me; that I wanted to shrink from the brilliance of the day like a vampire from the light by crawling into a box and hiding until the darkness came again. I wanted to say that sometimes, I had to remind myself to breathe—suck in and down and out consciously—using my mind to force my body to work when it didn't want to. I wanted to admit that now and then, my eyes felt like balls of cold mercury, pulled back into my skull by the weight of what they didn't want to see. I wanted to say that there were days when I clamped my hands over my ears to drown out the din of everyday noises that rang around my head like a kitchen full of children banging wildly on iron skillets with metal spoons. I wanted to tell Bert that I sometimes dreamed of my body, toe tagged, sitting unattended on a gurney, naked, white, exposed and not going anywhere because no one wanted to touch me. That other days, my head hurt, my heart felt numb, I couldn't smell, there was strange electric tingling in my hands and feet, my extremities went cold, my appetite disappeared and the only thing I wanted in the whole world was for someone to wrap their whole warm body around me and hold me. I wanted Bert to know that sometimes I was afraid to drive my car for fear that I'd intentionally drive into something—just to feel anything different than the feelings that always lurked below my determined, smiley public face.

Instead, I said, "Well, sometimes I do have difficult days."

Within several visits, I was a total convert to the powers of acupuncture and, specifically, to Bert. Simply by taking my various pulses and poking at my stomach, Bert could discern where I was weak—and make me stronger.

I lay on his table—a pale porcupine—breathing in rhythm to the nearly painless insertion of the needles. Especially when they went into places like under my pinky toenails, I wondered whether it was really necessary. But when he slipped needles under the skin on the insides of my bony knees—three inches of a hair-fine steely glint probing for a blockage in my energy flow— and my whole body sung with the sensation of released energy, I doubted no more.

During one of my visits, he placed a large stone on the middle of my chest. He left me to process. As I lay staring at the ceiling, tears started crawling down my temples. They came slowly at first, then faster, until I had strange, salty rivers burning the delicate skin on either side of my eyes. Because I was laden with needles, and the needles on my hands and those on my feet were connected with metal-clip-tipped ion pumping cords, I couldn't wipe the sadness from my face.

When Bert came back in, I apologized for crying.

"That is what's supposed to happen. The stone is a Native American technique for removing grief from your heart," he said.

It shocked me that not a single upsetting thought had crossed my mind and yet, I had bawled, without overtly thinking sad thoughts. It showed me how deeply I had stuffed the despair of my diagnosis and my fear of what would happen to me at the end of my life.

Bert taught me that when you really accept that you are going to die no matter what you do, life is a rich pageant indeed.

Had I truly embraced the idea of death? It was hard to say, because although I understood I harbored a life-threatening retrovirus, I looked and felt 100 percent healthy. So though I believed intellectually that death was coming, it remained an abstraction; something I could not feel to the point of real fear.

Just in case, and perhaps to stave off the onset of death by not denying its possibility, I planned the details of my funeral over and over again in my head. I hoped my imaginary construction of the event would somehow allow me to come to terms with my demise. I made a guest list, realizing that unlike a wedding, with a funeral you can invite people who don't get along. You can invite anyone you want. You're not going to be there to feel people's wrath or be stuck in the middle of awkward conversations; when you're dead, for Chrissakes, you can get away with anything.

*   *   *

Just as I introduced new rituals into my life, like acupuncture, and obsessively planned my final exit, I renewed old traditions, to connect with my favorite parts of my life. One of those was hunting for treasures at the flea market. Since I was in high school, my mom and I had spent glorious fall and spring mornings at the Golden Nugget flea market just outside of Lambertville, New Jersey. We played a game in which we wandered the lanes of junk trying to find the most remarkable object. Once we'd spied a contender, we'd drag the other over to it and indicate with raised eyebrows. It could be a bedraggled troll doll with a shock of electric green hair or a pair of gold brocade shoes with toes that turned up at the autumn sun or even a person, like the transvestite who worked at the vegetable and nut stand and liked to wear a sparkly bikini top even on days when you could see your breath.

One morning, I found a giant wagon. It was parked at the end of a lane and had great spoked wheels wrapped in bands of metal that had been worn smooth by miles of rolling over rock-strewn dirt roads. Once it had been painted bright fairground colors; when we saw it, the colors had faded to a pale patina.

"What is that?" my mother asked a man in a folding chair beside the wagon.

"It's a circus cart," he said.

A voice behind us whispered over my mother's shoulder, "It's a gypsy funeral cart."

We both turned to see the woman who was pointing at the faded caravan. She had a wild undone nest of gray hair and wore a dress that dragged in the gravel. She looked, like someone who could accurately identify a gypsy funeral cart. I smiled at her. She didn't smile back. She nodded, then walked away.

My mom looked at me, then at the cart. I could tell she

could see my mind turning. She was right: I pictured myself being dragged to my final resting place on that cart, pulled by piebald horses with feet the size of dinner plates. I could practically hear the sad, slow accordion music filling the air. Watching my mother's face—smiling on the surface and tense beneath—I could tell that she wasn't ready to start organizing my funeral procession.

"How much is it?" I asked.

"Eight hundred dollars," the man said.

Too much even for an indulgent departure.

We walked away and continued our morning's hunt, but I couldn't stop thinking about the mysterious rig and plotting the details of my demise.

My rendition of it changed all the time: the list, the location, the weather I hoped for, the music, whether I wanted people to laugh, or cry, or do both. After much contemplation, I was sure of one thing: I did not want to die, turn yellow or gray or green or whatever combination of colors you turn when the blood stops moving through your veins and the spirit has left your body, and have someone try to re-create, with waxy makeup, the way I looked when I was alive by rosy-ing up my cheeks or painting a lipsticked smile on my rigid lips. I wanted to be burned until there was nothing left of my corpse that could trap my spirit.

I want my ashes to be mixed with glitter (some blue, gold, green and rust) and multicolored sprinkles (the candy jimmies that go on top of ice cream). I want the whole sooty, sparkly, confection-flecked mix to be stirred, then spread over some emerald fields where horses roam and eat grass and where the land is open to the elements so I can dissolve back to the earth without a trace—save for some lonely specks of glitter that will catch the light, reminding any who visit the field of my passing.

*   *   *

The night after we found the cart, I heard the forlorn bellowing of young cows and bulls that were being weaned from their mothers. It was an early spring night, and the windows were open. The plaintive cries of the calves as they jostled, parentless, in the tight confines of the weaning pens, carried across the fields to my bedroom.

I lay in bed, remembering the primal sound my mom made when I told her I had HIV. Hearing the calves bawl for the warmth and familiarity of their mothers made me feel a sadness I realized that I had not yet allowed myself: though my mother was afraid and upset at the thought of losing me, I was equally petrified at the thought of having to lose her, too.

As the little cows wailed until they had no more energy to complain, I cried the tears that I had rarely allowed myself in the months since my diagnosis for fear that letting down my guard would lead to a fatal implosion. The sad calves pushed me over the edge of control. Grief that had been trapped inside of me like a wild animal in a steel cage hurled itself around my heart, struggling to get free. I buried my face in my pillow so Frank and my mom wouldn't hear me. I felt such guilt for making them worry about me every day; keeping my proverbial chin up, I thought, would lessen their hurt. But being unable to share my agony sawed at my chest and made me feel a loneliness so deep I felt like the only person who'd survived Armageddon.

In the months that followed, as the date of my expected death loomed, the pain of my emotional isolation grew unbearable— nearly as lethal as the virus itself. Many days, I felt like those calves bellowing across the night—terrified and incredulous that I'd been inextricably separated forever from a life that had once been happy and safe.

CHAPTER
seven

After many phone calls, my mother had gotten me an appointment with Dr. Cooper, one of the best AIDS doctors in the country. He was actively involved in research and worked at a university hospital in an inner city—somehow, my mom had convinced him to agree to make room for us in his busy schedule. And so, my mom and I climbed into her Volvo and went together to see the famous doctor.

We drove from Princeton to Philadelphia, parked the car and walked slowly into a waiting room full of cadaveric people who had AIDS—sticklike people with knees and elbows that protruded like doorknobs. They wore turbans and wheeled IVs behind them on spooky, screechy wheels. Some sat in wheelchairs. Some could not sit up. I took a huge gulp of air and perched on the edge of a plastic seat.

Because we were so far away from home, we weren't worried about running into anyone we knew.

My mom sat reading her novel until she couldn't pretend not to look around the room anxiously anymore. She was a nervous wreck, as was I, though she did the best she could to conceal her terror—both for my sake and the sake of those who waited with us.

To relieve some tension and make the time pass quicker, she asked if I wanted to play Hangman. At the time, it didn't occur to me how macabre her suggestion seemed. I was so eager for any distraction from my fear that my body would soon resemble the bodies of the people around us that the irony of her suggestion escaped me. We played for an hour until they called us in to see the doctor.

My favorite word she picked was "IV" It took me nearly twenty minutes, and the whole alphabet, to get it right. When I finalized realized what the word was, I screamed it out loud, "Oh, IV!" Then, horrified that those around the room hooked up to IVs had heard me, I stared nervously at the floor. I wondered whether she noticed, as I did, the awful similarities between the people in the waiting room and the stick figures we drew, hanging from the wooden gallows on the page. And whether she thought, as I did, that there but for the grace of God went I.

When my name was finally called, Dr. Cooper invited my mother and me to take a seat in the exam room. He introduced himself and told us to make ourselves comfortable—as if that was possible. He sat on a plastic chair with his legs spread apart. My mom and I sat side by side facing him. The exam table was ominously empty. He asked us why we were there.

"I was recently diagnosed with HIV," I said, trying to speak with confidence.

"How long ago?"

"About four months."

"Are you on medicines?"

"Yes," I said. My mother pulled a piece of paper from her purse and handed it to him.

baby through childbirth, or via breast feeding, and then there's the issue of getting pregnant without infecting your partner."

Sex. Could I have it? That's all I wanted to know.

As if he read my mind, he said, "You can have sex, as long as you use a condom. And theoretically, you could always get pregnant with the help of a turkey baster."

My mom looked like she might faint. She clasped and unclasped her hands in her lap. God, how could I have done this to her? I hated myself for putting her through this. I decided to change the subject.

"What about women dying sooner than men?" I asked.

"It's not that women necessarily die sooner than men," he said. "Men are just more likely to be diagnosed with AIDS. The reason for this is that fewer doctors look for signs of HIV in women and it often gets missed until it has caused AIDS, so they often have less time between their diagnosis and death. Many doctors, unfortunately, don't believe they should look for HIV in women. Because we only saw images of gay men with AIDS in the early days, a lot of people, including doctors, think it doesn't affect everyone, but I assure you, it does."

Judging from the diversity represented in his waiting room, he was clearly right.

"Let's do your blood work and see what we find," he said.

He called in a nurse who tied a piece of rubber tubing around my upper arm and drew my crimson blood into a series of glass vials. As the ruby liquid filled each one, my heart pumped a little harder with hope. This blood could show me that I had a future after all.

The doctor said he'd call us when he got the results of the blood work and recommend a new regimen of pills for me. I told him I'd love to have some new pills; the ones I was taking made me feel like there was a swarm of bees in my head. Dr. Cooper said that the new pills, taken as a "cocktail" or multidrug combo, wouldn't make me feel so sick. After we left his office, my mom and I drove in silence for a while. I waited for her to say something positive, or say that everything was going to be all right; but that wasn't what I was feeling.

I felt a clawing sense of isolation eating away at my insides.

Because I had HIV, I would be deprived of the comfort and support that people facing other deadly diseases received. The absence of my mother's comforting words after we left the doctor meant it was going to be up to me to summon the energy and vigor and cheer to constantly assure others that all would be well. It wasn't her fault. We were both experiencing emotional whiplash from going so suddenly from hopelessness to a place of tentative belief in a different outcome. While I understood why she didn't gush with enthusiasm, I wanted to punch someone, thinking about how goddamn unfair it was. If I had breast cancer, it would be so different. I looked over at her in the driver's seat, her pretty painted mouth set grimly in parallel lines—compressed to conceal an emotion I knew I didn't want to see. I sat in my seat, feeling like curling up like a spider, dying.

As we made our way through the chaos of Philadelphia and onto the main highway back to Princeton, I thought about a friend of mine from New Jersey with breast cancer, and how each time she went to her chemotherapy appointments, her mom took her for a celebratory ice cream on the way home. I wanted to ask my mom if we could stop at White Castle, or maybe the outlet shopping center, but I could tell that she wanted to get the day over and put it behind her as fast as possible. There would be no flowers, balloons or shopping sprees to celebrate my ongoing survival.

I went back through each moment of our visit, alternately

considering the experience from my perspective, and then my mother's. Had we felt, or heard, or thought the same things? I was so grateful that she'd come with me; what if I'd imagined the whole part about the new drugs being effective? Did the doctor really say I could have sex? Picturing every gesture and detail of my doctor's presence, I recalled how he had sat with legs sprawled out, directly across from both of us, while I was looking at other things to stare at besides his kind, penetrating eyes. It had taken considerable concentration not to study the strange bulge I noticed in the crotch of his too-tight khakis. I wondered if my mom had seen that, too. When he sat down, he yanked his pants up so they gathered in billowing folds of khaki around his pelvic area. I wondered whether it was air that bulged out his pants, or something else. Before that day, I would never have dared bring up such a topic with my mom. After discussing the salient details of my sex life in front of her, though, all bets were now, I imagined, off.

I decided to see if this was true.

"Mom . . . did you notice that the doctor seems to have unusually large . . . well, testicles?" I asked, suppressing my laughter at the word.

She said nothing at first; perhaps she was checking in with herself to see if she'd allow the new openness we'd established in the doctor's office to continue.

"Well," she said, a smile spreading reluctantly on her mouth. "It did look like he did have rather large . . . balls."

The idea of my hyper-polite mother saying the word "balls" out loud was too much. And, fueled by all the pent-up frustrations, tensions and fears that our trip to the doctor had engendered, I laughed, louder and louder, until I sounded like a hyena on helium.

She joined in and soon we were going back and forth like two kids.

"Doctor Big Balls!" I screeched.

"My, doctor," she said in a funny, low voice I'd never heard her use. "What large balls you have."

"My, are those balls big!" I squealed.

"*Very* big balls!" she said.

We meant no disrespect. The man had given me a second lease on life. But it just felt so damn good to release the terror and the darkness. And I loved my mom all the more for indulging in this highly uncharacteristic humor.

Before I knew it, my mom was pulling into White Castle after all, celebrating the fact that we'd survived our maiden voyage to the AIDS doctor, and believing, for the first time since we'd spoken of the disease, that maybe my survival was possible.

We got home and burst into the house, excited to tell Frank what we learned. He was elated for me. I called my dad and my sister and we all breathed a collective sigh of relief. It was amazing how the smallest dose of hope buoyed up my darkened soul. Spirited and reenergized, but always the pragmatist, my mother reminded us all that we didn't want to get too for ahead of ourselves. There was still the matter of waiting for my blood work.

I skipped through the rest of the day, feeling strong and ready to test my newly resilient body. I even went for a run. But when the sun went down, I found myself alone in my room envisioning what my life would be like going forward. Since my diagnosis, I had given up on falling in love again, and now, even if what the doctor said turned out to be true, the prospect of having more time felt bittersweet without a man to share it with. He'd said I could have sex with a condom, but all the steps I'd have to take before I could even worry about the whole condom thing overwhelmed me. Dating meant I'd have to tell more people about my status. Contemplating whether I'd have to spend the rest of my years alone, it was harder to feel happy.

Unable to sleep, I started poking around my room to see what remnants of my former life remained. Reaching under the bed, I found a relic from my childhood—my Barbie Dream House. When she left my old house, my mom had brought some pieces of our past with her. I dragged it out from under the bed by its handle and opened up the plastic mansion, releasing a smell as distinctive as bacon. It was all there, just as I'd left it in my other bedroom nearly two decades ago. Ken and Barbie were lying peacefully side by side in outfits that were one part *Hawaii Five-O* and one part *Austin Powers*. Barbie had on red velvet thigh-high boots and a tiny cotton smock emblazoned with fiery hibiscus flowers. Her golden tresses were piled on her head; a few tendrils hung down sexily across one eye. Ken wore light blue terry cloth shorts, brown rubber huaraches and no shirt. They were perfect, in face and figure. It was no wonder between playing with dolls like these, watching *Josie and the Pussycats* and obsessively reading *Vogue* that at 5 feet 8 ½ inches and 120 pounds, I thought my butt was big when I was a teenager. With HIV, I was never going to be like Barbie, my butt notwithstanding. And forget about finding my own Ken. I couldn't imagine a man who'd be capable of risking his life just to have sex with me, only to watch me die.

WINTER 1997–WINTER 2001

CHAPTER
eight

Dr. Cooper recommended that I see Dr. Giovanni, a great AIDS doctor in New York City, for my regular checkups, as he was so much closer. Dr. Giovanni looked like Gregory Peck, and his Upper East Side office was decorated like the Fifth Avenue apartments of many of my friends' parents. On my first visit, after we took care of all of the medical issues, he suggested that I allow him to introduce me to another of his patients, as a potential date.

This man was also HIV-positive, and a straight white lawyer living on the West Coast. I didn't even see a picture of him before agreeing to our having lunch together; if nothing else, I thought, it would be good practice at dating again.

I met George in the city and we got along really well. And I was attracted to him. He'd contracted HIV from his girlfriend, who'd used IV drugs. When she'd gotten very sick, the two of them sailed around the world in a sailboat until she died. That was a few years before we met and he said he was ready to try to find love again. We laughed, and talked, and he offered to come out and see me the next day in New Jersey.

I told my mother and Frank about my new friend and they said it would be fine to have him visit.

He took the train out from the city and I picked him up and made the short drive from the Princeton station to my mom's house. We all sat around for a while, making nice conversation and then, to have privacy, he and I went up to my room. Never, when I'd lived at home as a child, had a guy ever come upstairs with me at my house. So it was weird for George to join me, sitting, because there was nowhere else to do so, on the edge of my bed.

Eventually, he kissed me. But I recoiled, as I just couldn't make out with my mom downstairs, and it was all going too fast, and I wasn't sure I was ready to date yet—let alone date an HIV-positive man. I was still getting used to living with the virus myself; I still had so many questions. I really didn't feel capable of handling my own health, let alone thinking of another person's well-being at the same time. But because of meeting him, I got a glimpse of what people might go through when considering dating me: Would anyone want to fall in love with a person with HIV and risk losing her?

George and I have stayed friends, to this day.

My dad had recently moved to a new farm that had a small house beside the larger one. So, after nearly a year of living with my mom and Frank, I thanked them for their hospitality and love and moved again into my own space. It was perfect; I had privacy but my dad stood guard a hundred yards down the driveway. As much as I loved living with my mom and Frank, it was a little humiliating to be living at home with my parents in my late twenties. And not that I was truly entertaining the idea of one, but living with my parents made it impossible to imagine a love life again. I certainly couldn't have brought anyone home, nor stayed out all night, without them worrying and wondering about me.

Shortly after moving to my dad's farm, depression moved back into my life, mostly because I was afraid of being alone forever. There were some days when it would take me hours to get out of bed, or off the couch. I remember one day when I sat for countless hours looking out the glass doors that opened onto the bucolic backyard, staring blankly at a small herd of deer grazing. Watching the dappled fawns flick their tails happily in the sunlight as they chewed their first grass of the season, I marveled at how I could feel so horrible in the face of such beauty and light.

I'd made it to the first-year anniversary of my diagnosis alive. Realizing my body hadn't failed me and might hang in there for some years to come, but still battling depression daily, I decided it was time to get back on the horse—in a major way. So I took a job as a working student with my childhood riding coach, Carol, who was originally from England and rode in international show jumping and Three-Day Eventing competitions for Bermuda. She had a training facility not far from my dad's house.

I'd known Carol since I was eight years old, when she rented the farm where I kept my first pony, and I had always aspired to train seriously with her. But it seemed really impractical to try to become a professional rider and my parents discouraged it, hoping, instead, that I'd leverage my education in a professional arena. It wasn't that they didn't think I could do it, or that they didn't think being a professional athlete was a legitimate endeavor—they were just afraid for my health. Riding at the upper levels is dangerous, and my parents didn't enjoy watching as I hurtled around courses, risking my neck.

But because my distant future had been called in to question, all of a sudden I had a license to follow my dreams. And my life was already in danger. All the reasons I couldn't justify for taking a job with low pay and high physical risk vanished in the face of HIV. The least I could do, as I suffered the dark fears of days to come, was to follow my bliss with each new sunup.

Spending my days on Andiamo's back, leaping without fear over anything that got in our way was amazing medicine. There was a moment, at one horse show, atop a steep hill on the cross-country jumping course, when I could feel Andiamo's heart pounding between my black-leather-booted calves. We were headed to the next-to-last jump and there were two options— a bench to the left and a coop to the right. In between them was a five-foot-high cedar tree. As we bounded up to the jump, I decided to let him choose which side he wanted to go over. He chose the middle—straight over the tree. I screamed as he launched us both into the air and suddenly, I felt just like I had when I first grabbed the dolphins' fins, more than a year before. We hung in the air, flying for a second, weightless. His front feet hit the ground with a thud and he shook his head in the bridle, pleased with himself. As we galloped to the finish line, I cried because I'd lived long enough to know that moment of simple, pure joy.

Besides bolstering me physically and emotionally, working at Carol's 24/7 left me no time for a social or love life—and I didn't have to explain my absence in either sector. People understood that I had put my personal life on hold, in the aftermath of my divorce, to explore another great passion.

Carol was as tough, and as loving, as a second mother. I didn't tell her about my status at first. Before I shared the news with her, I wanted to prove to myself and to her that my HIV-positive body could handle the stress of mucking endless stalls and grooming and riding five to nine horses a day.

Carol's firm guidance and perfectionism when it came to the horses had made a deep impression on me. I greatly cared about her opinion of me and was terrified of displeasing her. So it was especially hard, when, after we'd been jumping one day and I'd nearly come off the horse midair, over a big oxer, I decided to tell her I had HIV.

I felt it was only fair; riding is dangerous, and if I fell and was bleeding, I wouldn't want her to touch me without taking the necessary precautions.

We sat in the office of her house surrounded by photos of her competing around the world. In many of the photos, a red, blue and yellow championship ribbon fluttered from her horse's bridle as she rounded the arena in a victory gallop. I stared at her strong, kind face under a sweep of thick brown hair. Her dark brown eyes watched me wearily; years of negotiating with creatures who didn't speak her language had sharpened her sixth sense; she knew something was wrong.

"Carol," I said, "I need to tell you something that may upset you."

"What is it?" she asked briskly in her clipped English accent.

"I hope it doesn't change the way you feel about me, but if it does and you want me to leave, please tell me," I said.

"What is it?" she said a little more insistently.

"I have HIV."

She didn't flinch.

"Thank you for telling me," she said. "It doesn't change the way I feel about you and I want you to continue to ride the horses."

I would have burst into tears of relief if I hadn't been so afraid to let her see me cry.

True to her promise, Carol didn't treat me any differently after she knew. She continued to drive me hard and expect the most from me, all the while feeding me the most beautiful home-cooked lunches and dinners, always making sure I ate my Brussels sprouts.

She refused to let HIV change our friendship or professional relationship, and her confidence in me made me grow stronger.

But the horses offered tenderness and an opportunity to nurture, too. My favorite part of the job was doing night check, wandering through the barns for a final time each evening, making sure the horses had enough hay and fresh water. I'd go into some of the stalls, to check whether a bandage was staying put, or whether a swollen leg had gone down. My final stop was always at Andiamo's stall. I'd turn over a bucket and sit by his front legs as I had that day we'd moved back to New Jersey together. He'd let his head sink down to mine, and he blew on my face and chewed on my hair. I told myself that this was all I needed.

Although my body seemed to be doing okay and I was tolerating well the drugs Dr. Giovanni had switched me to, and although the horses had helped me regain some of my effervescence, deep down I felt emotionally worse than ever since finding out I was HIV-positive. I couldn't understand it.

I went to see Dr. Giovanni in New York City and told him that I was struggling.

"This is going to sound really strange," I said. "But I think I'm depressed that I'm going to live."

The doctor folded his arms across his perfectly tailored suit and nodded.

"It's not strange at all," he said. "A lot of my other patients are going through the same thing."

He told me that many of us who had prepared as best we could to die were struggling with reorienting our minds and our lives to prepare to live. Rather than feeling unified with the community of other people who had HIV, or who had died from it, we were now disjointed—part of a new generation whose lives might be spared. And the result, while it should have caused relief, instead caused anxiety, and in many a phenomenon called survivor guilt. Why should we get to go on when so many just like us had not?

I didn't realize I'd done such a good job convincing myself that it was okay to die.

And it was strange to have lived through a year of acute drama, when my whole family was focused on my happiness, wellness and survival, and now to be living in a new era of their response to my diagnosis. The pain and worry of the first year had been so unbearable for all of us, but now the pendulum had swung in the other direction. It wasn't that any of us thought things would definitely be okay; we were just too tired of thinking they wouldn't, so we lived in a strange limbo of denial where we rarely referred to my disease. Part of me was grateful for the reprieve; part of me wanted them to send me flowers and a get-well card.

Don't get me wrong—I was grateful that I might live after all. But I was confused, and exhausted from the near miss. And, perhaps worst of all, no one could definitely tell me I was going to be okay.

Dr. Giovanni prescribed a mild antidepressant that made it possible for me to get off the couch with ease. Not because I was happy, but because the drugs removed all intense feeling. I wasn't sad anymore, but I wasn't happy, either. I felt as if I had a fishbowl filled with clear gel over my head. Sound, light, imagination, fear, lust, hunger, heartbreak—they all bounced right off the glass, leaving me staring blankly at them from faraway in my prison.

The antidepressant was good for my concentration and even eliminated some of the fear I felt when galloping up to big jumps on fresh unruly horses. But I missed the depth of feeling I had those first summer nights at Carol's when I sat with Andiamo, telling him the things I was afraid to express to anyone else.

Though I didn't like the numbness, it was better than the terror and apathy I'd known before.

So, two years passed at Carol's seemingly in a heartbeat.

One day, when summer was ending, and I thought of fall turning to winter and imagined months of getting up at six in the mornings in subfreezing temperatures, I questioned whether I wanted to stay. I loved riding, but I couldn't picture myself mucking stalls at forty. And with the help of the antidepressant, my strange sadness about survival was gone.

My time at Carol's had come nearly to its natural end; I had proven my mettle to myself, and I was ready to start planning for the long haul again. Working with Carol had restored my physical and mental well-being. I felt strong and tough. The combination of the news that I might survive and the help of antidepressants had finally allowed me glimmers of happiness. There were even days when I forgot about AIDS altogether—until I had to take my pills. Without even realizing it, I had begun living, not merely surviving. Though a part of me never wanted to leave the happiness of Carol's farm, I wanted my weekends back. I fantasized about maybe even trying to go on a date.

Almost as soon as I put that thought out to the universe, on one of the few nights I'd socialized in the two years since I had started working at Carol's, I met Charlie, who would later become my second husband.

Shortly after I told Carol I would be reducing my schedule, a former co-worker suggested that I come to a dinner party he was hosting. As it turned out, the party ended up happening at my house. While the early arrivals were having cocktails, Charlie pulled up in his red Saab, and emerged wearing low-slung jeans, cowboy boots and a suede jacket.

He had brilliant blue eyes and dirty blond hair. He was tall, and very fit from participating in triathlons. He had an easy smile and kind eyes. He was clearly used to the attention of women, but that didn't faze me; I paid no special attention to him throughout dinner, and I think partly because of my apparent indifference, he stayed after the other guests left.

His mother had been my field hockey coach at Princeton Day School; I'd known his younger brother Peter, who died, tragically, of a heart attack after waterskiing one summer day in the Adirondacks. Though I didn't really know Charlie, I knew his family, and he was from my world. When we met, he was living at his parents' house while they were in London, and I was still at my dad's. Our relationship progressed at lightning pace—perhaps both of us feared we wouldn't have much time together. I was far from convinced that I would live a long time, and he knew all too well how people he loved could be taken suddenly from the planet.

I was astonished to find love so easily after allowing myself the possibility of it again. At first, I'd been afraid that no one be with me because of the HIV, but Charlie seemed unafraid. He came to Dr. Giovanni with me in New York City and learned all about HIV. Once he'd absorbed the information and made his decision that the risk was minimal, we almost never discussed it again.

While we were dating, Charlie would wake up at six in the morning, make me coffee and turn on my car so it would be warm for my drive to the barn. He supported my love of riding; he even came with me to the Virginia Horse Trials, helping me lug bucket after bucket of warm water to bathe Andiamo in the crisp fall breeze after we came off the jumping course. Charlie met us at the finish line and we celebrated by drinking cold beers on hay bales as the rain that had made the hillsides slick thundered on the roof of the barn. I believed again in happiness.

I was grateful then, as I am now, for all Charlie brought to my life—especially at a time when I felt unlovable and lost. It would take another book to mine the intricacies of what made it all fall apart a year and a half after we got married, but suffice it to say that I was stunned to find myself packing my belongings and moving out of the farm we'd bought together, finding myself, at thirty-three, starting my life over, for the third time.

When Charlie and I decided to split up, I asked a family friend, Bryce, if he'd have me as a tenant above the old barn on his five hundred-acre farm. He said "of course," though he wondered out loud if I would really want to live in such a rustic place.

The barn had minimal baseboard electric heat and a wood-burning stove. The wind blew right through the cracks. It had been used primarily as a summer apartment for Bryce's polo pros. I wanted to be in a space with no distractions where I could process the reasons why I had been so unsuccessful at marriage. I had loved being married, actually. And I could imagine it working, with the right man, at the right time. Whether I married Andrew partially to overcompensate for the dissolution of my parents' marriage, and whether I married Charlie to fly in the face of my fears that I wouldn't have a future, I'm still not sure. I can say that when I agreed to marry both of them, it was with a sincere heart and a deep desire for a lifetime coupling. But there has always been in me a profound romanticism and an unwillingness to settle for anything less than a great love. When our love was forever tainted in both situations, I had to go.

The barn was unfinished and cavernous—just the kind of cave I needed to hide in, to go on a journey of self-discovery. It was the kind of place where I could write, walk in the woods, ride my horses, and be by myself in peace. I said I'd take it.

Being on Bryce's farm reminded me of living at my dad's. I would be in solitary confinement, but near people I trusted who could protect me. And I could bring the horses with me, and surround myself with nature.

As I rolled into the long stone-paved driveway the day I moved in, a horse and rider cantered along the grass airstrip that ran the length of the farm. The rider directed her horse to a jump and they sailed over. She leaned forward and stroked her mount's neck. The vision of the happy horse and rider was an omen that I'd come to the right place to find the parts of me I'd lost pursuing my completion through a man.

My years of riding taught me the importance of getting up again after falling off, brushing the dirt off my ass, and climbing back on the horse. I saw a bumper sticker I loved at a rodeo. It said: ARE YOU GONNA LIE THERE AND BLEED OR ARE YOU GOING TO COWBOY UP?

There was no way, after surviving two divorces and HIV, that I was just going to lie there and bleed.

SPRING 2002–FALL 2005

CHAPTER
nine

Shortly after I met Charlie, while I was still with Carol, I saw a copy of a glossy new lifestyle and design magazine called *New Jersey Life* and called to see whether they were looking to hire people. They were; I interviewed with the owner and publisher, a woman named Cheryl Olsten. Cheryl was beautiful inside and out with stunning chestnut hair, a quick wit and one of the most discerning senses of aesthetics I have ever known. She also rode horses.

Once I decided that I wouldn't make riding my whole life, I had started thinking about getting back into publishing. I missed writing, and the proposition of getting paid again to use my mind instead of my body was a welcome one. Riding is one of the toughest mental disciplines I have known, but my body was ready for a rest.

Cheryl hired me to be the magazine's managing editor, and eventually its editor in chief. We worked together for seven years making a lavish monthly magazine focusing on food, fashion, design, architecture, cars, jewelry, spas, gardens, animals and people.

I was in heaven being behind a desk again, spending my days pushing words around the page and organizing photo shoots of

life's most lovely things. We'd scour the faces of women, looking for the perfect one to grace our cover. Packages would arrive
containing tens of thousands of dollars' worth of exquisite jewels
or shoes or hats or garden accessories, and we'd get to see the insides of astounding homes and walk through secret gardens. We
discovered amazing wines and new swank restaurants and pried
recipes from the state's greatest chefs.

Under Cheryl's tutelage, I refined my eye and my sensibilities
as a magazine editor. And, I nearly forgot the ugliness of living with
HIV and put the discomfort of my broken marriages behind me.

Our offices were in a beautifully refurbished house in downtown Lambertville; my commute back to Bryce's was a mere fifteen minutes. Which meant that I had plenty of time to ride
Andiamo (I had, by that time, sold Milagro).

On my evening ride about nine months after I moved to
Bryce's farm, I noticed a car slow down and turn into the driveway while I was cantering Andiamo in circles on the polo field in
the front of the farm.

A blond man in his forties behind the wheel of a white Mer-
cedes inched tentatively toward me. He parked beside the ex-
panse of freshly mown grass and I thought as Andiamo and I
trotted toward his car that he was going to ask me for directions.
Instead, he said, "I'm so sorry to disturb you. It's just that I've
seen you riding around here on my way home from work, and
I've been wanting to introduce myself for a while. I'm Rob."

He was handsome in a weather-hewn way; his strong features
had been softened by the elements.

Surprised but intrigued, I hopped off Andiamo's back and,
lifting the reins over his head, took a step toward the car. "I'm
Regan," I said, smiling cautiously.

He got out of his car and offered his hand. It was warm and strong
as he held on to my hand for a few minutes. Letting go, he reached

out to give Andiamo a stroke on his neck, but Andiamo stepped quickly away. Rob laughed awkwardly and said, "I spend most of my time on the water; I've never really been around horses."

He explained that he'd recently moved to the area, owned a photography studio in Manhattan and had bought a farm not too far away. And after forty-five minutes of disarmingly comfortable conversation, he asked me whether I'd join him for dinner sometime. I told him, in a moment of boldness, that I would. I had been on my own for nine months; prior to that, Charlie and I had been estranged for a while. It seemed like forever since I'd had any romantic interest. My libido was slow to ignite, like the pilot light of a stove that's sat idle for a long time.

He asked for my number and typed it into his cell phone, got into his car and drove away. I hopped back onto Andiamo and, feeling weightless, lightly touched my heels to his sides, gave him his head and let him gallop freely down the polo field toward the barn.

Untacking Andiamo and putting him away, I thought about where Rob might take me, and what I might wear. I was so excited at the prospect of going out to dinner with a hot guy that I nearly forgot the terrible truth of my disease—and that I'd have to share it with Rob if we were going to date. It had been years since I'd had to face the issue of disclosure; I'd forgotten what a dark cloud it held over romance—at first. Imagining that when I disclosed to Rob he'd lose my number on purpose, all my joy evaporated.

I also worried about making Rob feel sorry for me. I worried about burdening him with the weight of my secret—I didn't want him to suffer by trying to respect my confidence but needing to talk to other people as he weighed whether or not to get seriously involved with someone who could get sick, make him sick, or die. I worried he'd tell someone. Or everyone. After all, I barely knew him.

He called the next day and we made plans for dinner that night.

As I got ready, I fought down a vicious depression. Dating is hard enough. Throwing HIV into the mix makes it immeasurably harder. Especially when you like someone enough to be afraid to disclose. And I really liked Rob. Would he be shocked when I told him that he'd fail to conceal his response? Would I be forced to see, firsthand, the unedited truth about what he thought about AIDS? I was terrified. Waiting while someone else figures out whether or not I'm worth the risk—of possibly being exposed to HIV, of falling in love with me, then having to watch me die from HIV, of maybe not being able to have a child or having a child with HIV, of having to lie to friends and family about the fact that I was HIV-positive—is agonizing.

You have to like someone to tell them or it isn't worth going through the discomfort. And liking them well enough to tell them makes the telling harder. With the telling comes the possibility of losing them. Tell them too soon and they won't be hooked enough on you to deal with the disease; tell them too late and they feel betrayed for falling for you, only to discover that you have a deadly disease.

Before I spilled the beans to Rob, I wanted to be sure that he cared enough to stay around long enough for me to give him the real skinny about HIV.

Otherwise, if he chose not to be with me, how would I know whether it was me, the virus, or something more basic that kept us apart?

When I walked into Rob's home, he had placed a bright burst of hot pink Gerber daisies on the kitchen counter for me. He couldn't have known, but I always said I'd marry any man who brought me pink Gerber daisies. I love their pop-art-colored petals, and I have always thought I could love someone who appreciated their cheerful simplicity more than the clichéd pomp and circumstance of a rose.

We had dinner at one of my favorite local country inns, laughing and drinking wine and alternately looking coyly and with mock defiance at each other. I felt, in some ways, like a total fraud, enticing him as I was without revealing my whole truth, up front. I quelled my concerns by telling myself he certainly had secrets that he wasn't sharing, either. Still, as few things seemed to be such an automatic deal breaker as telling someone you have HIV, I felt dishonest.

After dinner, when we were sitting in the quiet of his farmhouse living room, our faces barely lit by a sliver of a moon, I told him. While waiting for him to speak, I thought about how the moon looks new each time, though we know it is the same, and how the telling of my secret also always feels so different, despite the fact that it's always the identical process: disclose; comfort; assure; apologize; try to display dignity, remorse, humility and courage, then clamp a hand on your knee and paste a brave smile on your face, trying to look as understanding as possible while the other person's mind works like an intestine trying to digest a piece of cork.

It took the spit from my mouth, the breath from my chest. "Rob, I have something to tell you." The words came out jagged and fast. "I'm HIV-positive."

He just stared at me with eyes that had gone frighteningly cold.

"Do you get angry?" he asked, finally.

There are times, I wanted to say, when it feels like I've fallen and I'm trying to get up, and the only thing I can reach to pull myself off the ground is a chrome pole. And I'm wearing latex gloves. Smeared in Vaseline. And it's raining. There are moments, I wanted him to know, when smashing every glass thing in the kitchen and jumping up and down on the shards until my bare feet hemorrhage like freshly slaughtered pigs would not suffice to distract me from the pain inside, when bashing my hand against the wall until my bones were broken into hundreds of small pieces would not provide sufficient therapy for my anger.

But I didn't say that. Because I was trying to be chipper. Normal. Worth the risk. If I was scared, he would be terrified. I had to remain calm in order to convince him to embark on the reasonably risky journey we were contemplating taking together. It was too early to get into the nitty-gritty information that would eventually allay his fears. So I tried to tell him, in the most normal voice possible, and without sounding desperate or that I was trying to convince him to be with me, that the transmission of HIV can be prevented.

In as cheerful a tone as I could muster, I said, "Well, you won't get HIV if we have protected sex. I mean, I'm not assuming we're going to, or were going to, have sex. But just so you know, you can be safe without having to wear Andromeda-Strain-esque gear." I continued, with forced levity and confidence, "We can still have fun, we could even likely have an HIV-negative child. My doctor says I probably won't get sick and die, at least not from this, at least not any time soon. He says that my lifespan could be normal." Normalcy was the only thing I could think of to counter the news I'd just given this man who hardly knew me but who now knew my deepest secret.

"It must be depressing," he said after a long while.

And suddenly, just like that, I saw him differently—as a person much older than I was who had never contemplated death or his mortality or his purpose for this go-round on earth or the wonderfulness of whatever time we have. Even though I was younger, thanks to HIV I understood life differently, and maybe more richly, than he did.

"Well," I said, "it is sometimes. But it has also made me appreciate life so much more." I told him the story of the day of my diagnosis and how I went home after the appointment at the doctor's and savored my pasta.

I told him I realized that when they gave me my diagnosis they didn't really tell me anything I didn't already know. I was always going to die and I always knew it—my diagnosis just took away my ability to deny the reality of death by pretending I would live forever. But at the end of the day, everyone must look down the barrel of a shotgun to know what I know now.

Sitting in faint moonlight that was starting to feel creepy, not romantic, Rob stared at me with an unreadable expression and so, nervous to fill the space created by his silence, I launched into a harangue about the molecular behavior of the virus. "Well, you see, it replicates and the medicines work to thwart that replication . . ." I babbled on about the politics around AIDS and its impact on the global economy until I was tired of his saying nothing back. All hint of romance was now officially gone. So I left.

That was it. I never heard from him again. I bumped into him once years later at the coffee shop and he told me he was getting married. I wanted so desperately to know what it would have taken to have him accept me and my virus but it was too late. While deep down inside I knew there was no point in agonizing over someone who didn't want to be with me, it still hurt. But for all the havoc the virus had wreaked, in some ways it served as a protective shield, keeping away those who did not love me enough, and who probably wouldn't have been right for me anyway.

*   *   *

Several months later, still numb from Rob's rejection and fearful that I'd never again find a man who could deal with the HIV, I let my friends talk me into going to a Halloween costume party.

True to my plan, I had spent most of the time alone since coming to Bryce's. Though I absolutely wanted to date someone, I knew I needed to resolve a lot of things about my past, and the virus, before I attempted to share myself—and my life—with someone else. What happened with Rob was proof positive of that.

The friends who invited me to the party were brothers; they'd worked on the restoration of one of the old barns on our farm all summer and we'd become buddies. They all lived together in a big house on the outskirts of Princeton.

Since I was a little girl, Halloween had been one of my favorite holidays. In a little joke to myself, because I was always rescuing animals, I dressed as Cruella de Vil, the puppy poacher from *101 Dalmatians*. But I was so rusty socially that I had to struggle to enjoy myself; while people danced and laughed with abandon, I had close conversations with the several people I knew—standing in the corner.

At the end of the night, as I headed inside to collect my coat, I had to squeeze past a man standing in the doorway. He was dressed as James Dean, about the same age as Dean was at the height of his stardom, and better looking. He asked me for a light for his cigarette. I desperately wished I was a smoker.

"No, I don't smoke," I said.

"Yes you do," he said, winking.

Normally, I would have rolled my eyes and walked away from a line like that. But partially because he was doing his best to speak to me in my native tongue even though it wasn't his, and because I didn't mind the gist of what he was saying, I smiled at him.

"Where are you from?" I asked.

"Ukraine," he said with a voice that felt like it was crawling around my body.

Forrest, as he called himself, was a professional soccer player who had come to the United States to be a model. The friends who had brought him from New York City to the farm in New Jersey where the party was had accidentally abandoned him and returned to the city.

"I don't have a car or a place to stay. Can I come home with you?" he asked in his low, heavily accented voice.

I'd never been propositioned so directly. I had no idea whether he simply needed a place to sleep or whether he wanted to sleep with me. I knew his friends who had brought him out from Manhattan, so it was unlikely that he was a sociopath. Further more, since I had no intention of being with him because there was no way I was disclosing my HIV status to some stranger whose trustworthiness and discretion I didn't know, it seemed okay to provide him with some innocent shelter. And stare at him a little.

When we got home, I went into the bathroom to remove my Cruella de Vil costume and makeup. When I came out, I couldn't find Forrest. I wandered around my barn and, going to the last place I expected to see him, discovered him lying naked on my bed. I had never before seen a body like that. He made the Abercrombie & Fitch guys look flaccid. I laughed nervously.

"Get up and get dressed," I said.

He stared at me incredulously and didn't move. He touched his inner thigh and flashed his teeth.

"I mean it," I said. "Please put your clothes on and go sleep on the couch."

"Why? You don't like this?" He rubbed his hand across his chest and down his stomach, looking down his aquiline nose at his twelve-pack.

"Yes I do. It's very nice. Very nice," I said. "But I want you to get out of my bedroom."

"No woman," he said with a confident smile, "has ever rejected me. Not once, on four continents."

"Well," I said, "welcome to America. Put your clothes on." And I tried pulling him by the hand off my bed. He yanked me down on top of him and tried to kiss me.

I wrestled free with perhaps more force than was necessary, causing him to storm around getting dressed and then sulk noisily on the couch. He made one more attempt to join me during the night; even half asleep and though some subconscious animal part of me wanted him to stay, I managed to thwart his final advance.

In the morning, I found him staring at the ceiling, looking totally despondent.

He'd taken my rejection to heart. To spare his feelings, and his ego, I decided to tell him the real reason I didn't want to touch his perfect body. When I told him I had HIV, he yelled something at me in Ukrainian and ran out of my house. I wondered where he planned to go, given that I lived on a five hundred-acre farm in the middle of nowhere and he had no car. I felt as rejected as he did—and I wasn't running around cursing in arcane tongues. It doubly pissed me off because my attempt to nurture his fragile ego had resulted in mine getting a body blow.

I peered out the window and watched him pace around gripping his gold tufts of hair with clenched fists.

Eventually, he crawled back up the stairs and sat on the couch staring at me. I told myself that he was just frustrated that he couldn't be with me. It wasn't true but it made me feel better.

We had some language issues but came to an understanding. Eventually, he saw that I really had done him a favor. I had protected him from himself. He came over and touched my cheek as a gesture of . . . I wasn't sure. But it felt good to feel his hand on me, good to be held, even if only by his fingers, lightly. It had been hard to turn away from such an offering, but looking at his near perfect, youthful beauty, I was proud of my restraint, glad for all those years of sexual discipline that had come in handy in the heat of the moment.

We went to Burger King while we waited for his friend from New York City to come and retrieve him. He asked a lot about the disease and me and my life and I learned a lot about professional soccer. Listening, I remembered being in Burger King with my sister that first day she and I talked about HIV. I noticed Forrest, unlike my sister, was careful not to dip his fries in my ketchup.

We eventually hugged good-bye and gave each other greasy kisses on the cheek. He promised to call, but I knew from the look on his face that I would never see him again. I was beginning to think that what seemed like a new and deep bond in the aftermath of disclosure was more about his relief from having narrowly averted sleeping with someone with HIV.

As I walked across the abandoned parking lot to my car, I had to jump at the last minute to avoid stepping on a dead bird on the roadside—an inert, black, shiny, sweet potato of a dead crow. Before I knew it, I had burst into hysterical tears. I couldn't bear the thought that he'd never again sit on a fence post in the morning sun, opening his wings to dry the dew between his feathers. I cried for all the worms he'd never eat, for all the aerial glory his downed body would never know. I know it was the anticipation of my own fallen self that I saw in him; I know that I cried for all the morning suns I feared I was going to miss, but I would not admit that to myself. To combat my depression, I went to the car wash.

The Shammy Shine on Route 31 lets you stay in your car. You

can drive nearly anything through the Shammy Shine. One time I went, a man pulled a small sailboat through behind his sedan. I don't like the car washes that make you get out and watch your car progress from dull to high gloss through the windows; it's just not as much fun as staying in your car, tilting back the seat, turning up the tunes waiting for the pastel confection of soap to Jackson Pollock your window. I love watching the Easter-colored droplets converge and melt down my windshield, washing my cares away. It was like sliding through a kaleidoscope.

The analogy of the car wash is simple: you go in dirty on one end and come out clean on the other. It's hard to feel filthy when your car is all sparkling glinty-clean and smelling lemony fresh. I like to pretend that the chute of pressurized jets of scalding water, spinning scrub brushes the size of oil drums and the happy soap is capable of sloughing off the viral particles clinging with a vengeance to my healthy cells. I find it helpful to picture my sickness getting a bath.

Besides the pretty soap and clean feeling there are also the attendants: flush-faced, doe-eyed, faux-hippie college boys— trustafarians—whose rich parents have insisted on summer employment. They move their oversized, flip-flopped feet around the wet tarmac with defiant insouciance, dragging their heels in protest at being forced to participate in the service industry.

There was one who seemed he might do more than abuse his inheritance. His step had an irrepressible bounce and his mouth was permanently on the verge of a smile in contrast to the forced, studied scowls of his co-workers. There was pressurized joy in him, like the air in a can of Play-Doh. It was rare that I would emerge into the bright flash of sun at the end of the dark tunnel without feeling better, but occasionally, when the spitting soap failed to make me smile, the sight of his pouncing walk dissolved the last traces of my creeping depression faster than the industrial-strength cleaning agents that took the road grease off the undercarriage of my car.

As he rubbed a chamois cloth over the nose of my car, he looked at me and curved his mouth. We would never know each other, never touch, never speak, never trouble each other's lives with fears or needs or insecurities or contaminated bodily fluids. Our connection was limited to the space and time just after my car emerged from the car wash shaft. His boundless energy as he polished away stray beads of water reminded me of a time when I believed there was a way out of every problem, or at least enough time left in my life to have even the most horrific problems dissipate to black nothingness. Now I knew that there were some things that would never fade in a lifetime. HIV threatened to overshadow my whole life, compromising the luster of it. And so I kept returning to the car wash to spit-polish my dampened spirit with candy-colored soap and boys who smiled flirtatiously at me because they did not know about the poison in my veins.

CHAPTER

ten

Though Rob couldn't handle my positive status, having had him express interest in me helped bolster the esteem that HIV, and my divorces, had taken from me. But I would be lying if I said his rejection, and Forrest's, didn't shake my confidence that a man would be willing to cope with HIV. So while I tried having a drink, or dinner, here and there, with a man who seemed interested in getting to know me, I spent the whole time wondering whether he seemed substantial enough to hear my truth, and in the end, I often couldn't speak it. My reservoir of resilience was empty; I told myself that I couldn't tell this man or that one because they weren't emotionally developed enough to handle my disease, but the truth was that I simply couldn't withstand another rejection. I had two brief relationships—one was quasi platonic, the other long distance—with two amazing guys. But again, whether because I believed it to be true, or whether it was real, HIV stood in the way of anything getting too serious.

Instead, I focused on my friendships with my girlfriends Courtney, Sally, Susie, Elizabeth and Jane, whom I'd befriended since moving to the farm, post-divorce. And I was thrilled to spend more time with my sister Tracy, who'd recently moved back to the area with Josh, who was now her husband.

We'd meet weekly at Ota Ya, the local sushi restaurant for Girls Night Out. We went so regularly that the waitresses stopped giving us menus because they already knew what we wanted. We'd stay until past closing, emptying bottle after bottle of wine, while the staff vacuumed around us. All of us were horse owners and riders, so there was a lot of horse talk—and, of course, a lot of talk about men. Every now and then, they'd try to set me up with someone they knew, and I'd balk because I didn't want to end up liking him, telling him I had HIV and worrying that he'd tell my friends.

It wasn't that I didn't trust my friends to hold my secret; I didn't want to burden them by asking them to hold it. And I didn't want them to worry about me, or pity me, or treat me any differently. Maintaining normalcy was very important to me as I tried to live as full a life as possible. How could I feel healthy and strong if people were concerned about me all the time? There were times when one of my friends would drink out of my glass, or kiss me good-bye on the lips after dinner, and I worried that one day, when I told them—as I eventually knew I would—that I had HIV, they would freak out, remembering how close they'd come to my virus. But by then I knew the truth—that those things didn't put them at the slightest risk—and I knew they would believe me someday when I told them. Mostly, I didn't tell them because I needed a safe place to go, hang out, drink wine, talk, laugh and pretend there was nothing wrong with me—other than the daily concerns we all shared about getting along with our families, finding a good hair colorist, finding homes for the endless litters of kittens born in our barns and finding happiness with our men.

*   *   *

I was having drinks with my girlfriends one spring night at one of my favorite riverside watering holes when I noticed a dark-haired man whose electric eyes stared directly into mine each time I glanced across the room at him.

I pointed him out and they craned their necks to catch a glimpse, but he'd disappeared. I remember feeling a jolt of electricity and then a deep disappointment that I'd missed the chance to talk with him. But I also felt a strange certainty that I'd see him again.

Several weeks later, I did.

I was having dinner with Courtney at the same spot I'd first seen him. We were deep in a conversation about how to keep Andiamo's four hooves on the ground—he had taken to rearing and bucking after each jump—when I noticed that the man was back. Sensing my distraction, Courtney looked over her shoulder and raised her eyebrow. As if knowing he was being watched, he stood up—he was tall, 6 feet, 3 inches, lanky and wore a black short-sleeved T-shirt over a long-sleeved undershirt, army pants and black Converse sneakers. He stretched his hands over his head to reveal a swath of bare stomach and sauntered past us to get another drink from the bar. He had an incredible head of thick, dark hair and a dark chocolate beard, and he was much younger than I was. His eyes were defiant and sharp as they surveyed the room. As he walked past, his eyes met mine and lingered in what felt like a challenge.

It was unnerving, but as much as I wanted to look away, I couldn't. I finished the meal, trying hard to concentrate on Courtney's suggestions for taming Andiamo's resistance while thinking how to start a conversation with my dark-eyed neighbor.

After dinner, as we slowly donned our coats, I feverishly hoped he would do or say something; he was sitting a mere ten feet away. I have been told that I can seem unapproachable, so as we passed his table, I paused and said, "Where did you get your tattoo?"

I had noticed before that he had a large black fleur-de-lis inked on the inside of his right forearm. In a circle around the symbol, heavy black text said: "Past Is Prologue."

Just after asking him, I realized that the other three young men at his table were also—and more intricately—tattooed; one had a large ship on his upper arm. It was as detailed as fine scrimshaw. My cover was blown—if it was tattooing that I'd really wanted to discuss, I'd have been talking to him.

Sensing my awkwardness, he smiled a little, introduced himself as Jody and told me that he'd gotten the tattoo locally. We fell into easy conversation. He asked what I did and I told him I was a writer. For the next few minutes, we chatted but the words were inconsequential—our eyes were locked together.

Courtney coughed to remind me she was there.

"I think I'm going to head out," she said with a mischievous grin.

"Okay," I said. "I guess I'll see you . . ." I trailed off awkwardly.

"Tomorrow," she said, smiling.

She left, and Jody offered me a seat.

He introduced me to his friends and we talked about music and fishing and dogs and wine and gardens and horses and books.

After about forty-five minutes, he asked if I was cold.

"Why?" I said.

"Because you're still wearing your coat."

I hadn't even noticed. No wonder my face was flushed.

Jody called the next day and again several days later and invited me to go for a walk with him along the river. And over the next couple of weeks, as we rocked on the porch of his dad's house, where he lived, we drank wine he brought home from the local wine shop where he worked. We slept together sometimes at his house, curled up on the floor with his husky, a two-toned dog named Juneau, or in the tree house in the giant sycamore behind his house and sometimes at my house, covered in the wild cats I'd rescued from the many litters born in the horse barn. Some nights, I'd sleep beside a fire with him at the river's edge and go straight to work.

Jody was fiercely principled and idealistic; he was the lead singer of a hard-core band called Fire Season. When he wasn't practicing, or helping people choose wine, he'd camp down by the river with his brother, Nick, and his friends, cooking Delaware catfish over an open fire, writing songs and discussing how we should all live differently than the modern world dictated.

Jody was a big fish in a small pond; with the exception of spending some of his college years in England, he'd never been far away from his hometown of Stockton, New Jersey. Everyone in town, of all ages, knew him. He was the kind of person you'd want beside you when life got complicated; he could diffuse the most volatile of situations with a handful of the right words and he always had thoughtful solutions to everyone's problems.

People listened to him, and he always had something helpful, challenging or inspirational to say.

His friends joked that he was like Peter Pan, and I was Wendy to his Peter and his friends, who were indeed a little like the Lost Boys. They all knew about my HIV; the way I'd dealt with it had earned their respect. They were all hard core—so was I, in a different way. We were a posse; fishing and canoeing and walking in the woods together, dreaming of changing the world, of living off the grid and outsmarting the machine. Though I kept telling myself that our own little utopia of openness, freedom and acceptance could be replicated in society at large, I knew, intuitively, that our togetherness was not sustainable. Often, it felt as if we were in a synchronization of time, elements and circumstances that would never again be replicated in our lives and, in its recognizable etherealness, was all the more precious.

I know it seemed weird to my friends and family that I was spending my time with someone so much younger, but having endured such grown-up pain for the bulk of my twenties, I relished living a carefree life with people who were still so young they thought anything was possible.

Jody wanted to leave a lasting mark on the world, and he wanted me to help him do it. We just didn't know, in the beginning of our time together, how that would happen.

When I told Jody that I was HIV-positive, he didn't fear the disease for a second. That was mainly because he knew so little about it. He hadn't been born when they first discovered the virus and he hadn't grown up, as I had, watching the horrific images of AIDS ravaging people all over the world. To him, it was merely a disease that could be managed and prevented. He was stunned that there was so much stigma around HIV and we had endless conversations about how ludicrous it was that HIV had the rap it did. He reasoned that people's discomfort with AIDS was tied to their discomfort with the notion of gay or anal sex and said it was ridiculous. He was the first one to tell me that when he was a teenager he knew a lot of young people who engaged only in oral and anal sex as a way to preserve their virginity. Anal sex, he assured me, was not the sole property of gay men. In fact, heterosexual tweens and teens were having it all the time.

We spent a lot of time on the Delaware River, having philosophical conversations as we slid down the slow-moving water in a canoe on many a Sunday afternoon. Other than our words floating over the water, the days were so quiet you could hear the flap of rooks' wings as they circled over the river. When the sun burned his shirtless back, Jody would slip over the edge of the boat like an otter, moving in a single pulse of a muscle, disappearing beneath the British racing green–colored water and pop his head up fifty feet away, shaking the water from his eyes with a quick jerk of his head.

He called his canoe *Bertha*; more than once I'd carried the oversized green craft up the hill to his house post-river journey complaining that because I was a good five inches shorter than Jode (everyone's nickname for him), I was doing most of the heavy lifting. It was the way most things happened between us. The sheer force of who he was kept him from seeing the power of his impact on other people, especially those who loved him and tried feverishly, as I did, not to disappoint his expectations of our abilities—our inherent greatness—as he saw it.

He always pushed me to consider my choices and sometimes to rethink them. He loved who I was but wanted me to be all he imagined I could be. He cajoled, shamed, encouraged and sometimes dared me to move beyond my comfort zone. All the time. Nothing was easy with Jode but being with him was always an adventure.

One day, Jody and I swam in the river when the water was low. Swinging from a rope tied to a tree, we pushed ourselves harder and harder so we could launch ourselves farther out to the deeper water. Then we waded slowly over the mossy rocks back to shore. As I traipsed through the water, he bent down and scooped a handful of mud from the river's floor and flung it onto my bare stomach. I threw some back at him and soon we'd thrown so much mud at each other that we were nearly indistinguishable from the brown of the water itself. Eventually, we waded to shore and walked through town, forgetting we were covered in mud, maybe looking to passersby like a strange pair of warriors from a more primitive time.

Of all the things Jody taught me, one of the most important was to face the things that terrified me. He was afraid of nothing. When I admitted that the secrecy of my HIV status was trapping me in a miserable, stomach-curdling pinch of fear, he suggested I address it by moving toward it, not away.

While I was working at *New Jersey Life,* before I met Jody, I had found a magazine called *POZ* at my doctor's office. It was for people living with and affected by HIV. Wanting to become involved in AIDS activism but still too afraid to come forward, I'd started writing a column for *POZ* under the "Anonymous" moniker. In each column, I'd disclose to someone and write about the experience of weathering their reaction. With each column, I got a little bolder and the writing got a little easier. It became more and more clear that the shame around HIV was not mine to bear, but rather should be borne by those who lacked the decency to understand the basic science of the disease and treat those living with it with dignity, regardless of how they contracted the disease or what their sexual orientation was.

As my friends still didn't know I was living with the disease, and because my family and I now only talked about it every three months or so when I'd share the results of my routine blood work with them, *POZ* was my only lifeline to a whole world of people living with HIV. With each issue I would stare endlessly at the pictures of the people on its pages and feel connected to them.

Each time an issue of *POZ* came, I'd show it to Jody and proudly point out my column.

Jody believed in acknowledging all truth and staring it down. He lived to daylight every insecurity, dragging it into the open, shaming ourselves into a place of total honesty which, he said, was the only truly safe place to be because then no one could pressure us to do anything we didn't believe in.

One day I realized that I'd been writing my column for *POZ* for almost four years and that I'd been living with HIV for nearly ten. And though I'd told an increasing number of people, the majority of people who knew me still had no idea I had HIV. *POZ* had recently given me a longer assignment, still under the moniker of "Anonymous." The piece was titled "Lines Composed in a Looking Glass." It was to be my first-person account of fearing that disease progression or the effects of my treatment would noticeably change my body and thus give away my tightly guarded secret that I was living with HIV.

I was worried that writing such a long and personal story would prove problematic.

Though I wanted desperately to take the plunge I still struggled.

On the same day I had been thinking about taking his suggestion of moving toward my fear of public disclosure, perhaps by putting my real byline on my articles instead of "Anonymous," Jody said, so bluntly I was stunned, "I'm having trouble committing to you because I'm worried you'll die before I do."

"But none of us knows when we're going to die," I protested, a chill creeping up my neck. This was his preamble to leaving my side.

"True, unless they have a terminal disease, like you do."

"Ouch," I said. "I have totally embraced the notion that I could live a normal lifespan, why can't you do that, too? Don't you remember what the doctor said?" I reminded him of the words he'd heard when he'd gone with me to my last checkup.

"Yeah," he said, "you might have a normal lifespan. But you're thirteen years older, and have HIV, so your life will be probably be shorter than mine."

In the end, he was dead wrong about that.

I was devastated. His contagious idealism and sense of invincibility were just what any good doctor would have prescribed for my fear of a premature death.

We ended our love affair at the Prallsville Mill, sitting in a car, watching the river flow by, carrying away all our dreams of a future together.

WINTER 2005–SPRING 2007

CHAPTER

eleven

On a rainy December night, while buying hay for the horses at a local farm, I got a strange call on my cell phone.

The man for whom I would eventually work introduced himself, said he had purchased *POZ* magazine from its founder, Sean Strub, and asked whether I'd be interested in interviewing for the position of editor in chief at *POZ*.

"I got your name from Walter," he said, referring to the editor in chief I'd written for over the past several years. "He's moved on and thought you might want to take his position at *POZ*."

The summer before, on mediabistro.com, I'd seen that the position was open. I'd briefly contemplated throwing my hat in the ring but didn't feel ready to disclose at the time. I'd settled down after my divorce from Charlie, and I loved working at *New Jersey Life*. I couldn't imagine blowing my life apart again so soon after I had pieced it all back together. But that night, as the rain washed the windshield and the winter wind howled around my car, I pulled over to the shoulder to talk.

I said nothing for a moment, watching the windshield wipers swing rhythmically across the glass. Something about their cadence, and the portentous feeling of this phone call, reminded me of the syringe swaying back and forth on its point on the day when I was diagnosed. I could feel my life changing again—seismically. I said gingerly to the man on the other end, "Sure, I'd like to talk with you about that."

We set a time to get together.

I had already achieved one of my career goals—I had become editor-in-chief of *New Jersey Life*. But as much as I loved the magazine and working with Cheryl, I had always dreamed of being a war correspondent, of writing stories about life—and death. Working for *POZ* would not make me a war correspondent. But it would take me back to earlier days, when I wanted to have an impact on people's thinking by doing groundbreaking stories on volatile and taboo subjects—and by writing about life, and death.

But I still seriously doubted whether I could withstand disclosing to the world. And I didn't want to hurt my family. Was it selfish, I wondered, to drag people I loved and respected through a host of painful consequences? Even if it meant that I could be open about what I was going through, and maybe even help people who were going through the same thing? The trade-off seemed fair; but I worried that the fallout would be too big to handle, that I'd wind up alone at holidays and sleep forever in an empty bed. As much as I cared about the unseen legions of people suffering with HIV around the world, and as much as I wanted to try to help them, I knew it would be hard to focus on relieving their pain if doing so caused my family to suffer right under my nose.

But before I dismissed the idea entirely, I decided to ask them what they thought I should do. What they wanted me to do. What they didn't want me to do. They'd surprised me with their supportive reaction to my status. Maybe they would be similarly supportive about the idea of my going public.

I did have some clues to how they felt. The Christmas before, I'd sent my mom, dad and sister a letter explaining some of my feelings about HIV that I'd never been able to express in person. The letter was part apology and partly a plea for help. For years we'd all tried to get our heads around my health crisis. Some days it seemed a thing of the past and some days seemed to define—and possibly steal—my future. By then we'd all developed AIDS fatigue. None of us wanted to talk about it, worry about it, pay for it, or fear it anymore. But though the treatment had decreased the replication of the virus sufficiently for my immune system to stay robust, and, for the most part, strong-arm HIV into submission, I was still not out of the woods. And the fear of being stigmatized still gnawed at my innards.

Frank, perhaps because we weren't blood related, was able to confront me after reading the letter, while the others in my family barely acknowledged it. In a rare act of directly involving himself in my life, he called and invited me to dinner at the local pizza place one night when my mom was out of town. At first, I thought he was just trying to deepen our relationship; or perhaps he was just looking for company.

Shortly after the waiter uncorked the wine, he pulled the letter I'd written from his pocket. Holding it between his thick fingers, he said that it had had a powerful impact.

"You should share these feelings with others," he said.

He explained that he had never known or thought about many of the things I wrote about in my attempt to let my family in deeper to my experience of living with HIV.

"You could help people if you could tell this stuff to the world," he said.

I said that I would certainly deeply consider doing so. I thought he might be right, but I didn't know if I had the strength.

After *POZ*'s owner proposed that I take the editorship, I had hours of conversation with my mom, my dad and Tracy. My mom was concerned about a lot of valid issues: whether I'd lose my friends or my housing, be ridiculed or ostracized. It is one thing to tell the people in your world that you are living with HIV; it would be something else to tell the world. Working for an AIDS magazine every day would bring AIDS into my life in a way I never imagined. And as the editor, I'd inevitably be constantly, and publicly, connected to my HIV-positive status, whether that meant being quoted or interviewed or appearing in person to speak about AIDS. I worried that I'd never date again: after I let my news out in such a public way, I'd never again have the chance to let someone get to know me before finding out I was HIV-positive. I wondered if I'd tire of devoting my whole life to AIDS; I'd have no future outside the field once I disclosed, and would therefore cast my lot permanently with the disease.

At first, my mom was hesitant to encourage me to come forward.

"You should think really hard and long about this," she counseled. "You won't be able to take the decision back."

It was hard for me when she didn't instantly leap to support any decision I made.

"I know you will help change misperceptions about AIDS, but I'm worried about the price you'll have to pay," she said.

And then I realized she was only being protective, as any mother would.

My sister Tracy shared some of my mom's concerns. But she thought I should do it.

"Whatever bad things people might think about your having

HIV," she said, "they'll overcome by respect, because you came forward to try to help people."

Interestingly, my dad thought I should absolutely take the job—for my health.

"It's not healthy to hold in a secret like this," he said. "Whatever happens, you'll be free from worrying, and that will make you feel better."

Though Jody and I weren't talking at that point, I thought about what he'd said before, when trying to entice me into full disclosure. "Keeping your secret is more dangerous to your health because of the stress that creates, than whatever harm comes from the things the world will do or say when you tell the truth," he said. "Plus, when you speak your truth, it shields you."

My own concerns echoed those of my family—and I had others as well. What if I couldn't handle the stress? And the HIV community, which in America had historically been composed of gay white men, might not accept me. Perhaps I was an outlying statistic, the kind that researchers throw out when trying to track viable trends; perhaps I didn't fairly represent who had HIV at that time. But then I visited the website for the Centers for Disease Control and Prevention and had my mind blown open.

It had been a long time since I'd seen the figures for who had AIDS around the world. When I scrolled through the data in 2006, I was shocked to discover that women comprised more than 47 percent of all infected people worldwide. In the United States, nearly a third of all people living with HIV were women. I looked at the numbers again and again, feeling a strange mix of emotions: on one hand, I was glad to discover that I wasn't a freak; on the other hand, I was horrified that awareness and prevention efforts had failed so miserably around the globe that the numbers of people infected with a preventable disease were exploding. Especially among people who might not have considered themselves at risk—women, African Americans, Latinos and young gay men.

When I was first diagnosed, I had read obsessively everything about AIDS I could get my hands on, including my doctors' textbooks. But after getting a good grip on the facts of AIDS, I took a break from studying the disease; in the years since then, much had changed. Until I pored over the latest facts, I hadn't realized how out of touch I was with the modern epidemic. AIDS had gotten more out of control than anyone had predicted.

I decided I would go for it. I had to. Once I had the support of my family, I didn't have anything else to lose.

First, though, I had to get the job.

POZ's owner and I had lunch in Princeton. Since the magazine had been bought by someone who was not HIV-positive and had no connection to the world of HIV, I feared *POZ* might lose its editorial integrity.

POZ was founded by Sean Strub, a gay man living with HIV, and it had always been an uncompromised platform for the collective voice of the HIV community. Diagnosed at the beginning of the epidemic, Sean had used a viatical settlement from his life insurance policy (knowing you are dying, you can cash in your life insurance early) to found *POZ* magazine.

He did so to try to ensure that all people in America with HIV would have access to the information they needed to save their lives. And that this information would be unfettered, free of the outside influences that all too often contaminate much of today's news and information. If that was even possible. Sean, and all who have worked with him at *POZ* from the beginning, proved it was.

When I had lunch with the new owner in Princeton, he told me that it would be my job to protect *POZ*'s legacy of empowering people living with HIV to advocate for and access the best health care.

The owner had me speak with Sean and after that, I met the whole incredible staff at *POZ*. Humbled, grateful and so excited, I called my family to say that if this group of people considered me worthy to edit *POZ*, I'd have to try.

I couldn't wait to tell Jody.

I went to his house for the first time since we'd broken up more than a year before. It was a frigid December night, and I'd bought him a book about extreme explorers. I wanted him to have it for his birthday, which was coming up on January 11. I sat at his small kitchen table petting Juneau as he made me one of his usual camping dinners of baked beans and bacon and scrambled eggs.

"Guess what?" I asked Jody.

"What?"

"I got the job of editor in chief at *POZ* and am taking it."

He stopped stirring the beans and turned slowly to look at me with a large, wolfish grin.

"I'm so proud of you," he said. He walked across the kitchen and took me in his arms. "You know that no matter what happens from this point forward, you've already gone past a point that most people will never experience."

I beamed at him and we thumbed through the book of explorers, talking about someday taking a journey together. He seemed so pleased that his influence on me had brought me to a place of light and happiness, and kept looking closely at my face while we read the book. He had started to call me again regularly and asked me to consider whether we could get back together. I told him life would have to work itself out, but that I would never say never.

Before I left, I confessed to Jody, "I'm so scared about whether I can do this."

"By just agreeing to try you are already a success," he said.

I told him I'd call him to let him know how my first day went. He kissed me long and hard and said he'd see me soon. But I never spoke to him again.

My first day at POZ was January 10, 2006, the day before Jody's birthday. I couldn't tell anyone besides my mom, dad, Tracy and Jody where I was going; we'd decided that I would "come out" as HIV-positive on my first cover—the April issue. So I worked in secret. Even just one day at POZ made me feel like a prisoner who had escaped from serving a life sentence. Everyone was so nice, and supportive. And while I loved the glamour of New Jersey Life, it was a welcome change to write about such meaty things as Congressmen blocking bills that would secure access to care for HIV-positive people, the latest HIV treatments and the travel ban that prevents HIV-positive people from entering the United States. Things that directly affected the quality and length of the lives of people living with the virus. After my first day, as I drove through the Lincoln Tunnel, heading back out to New Jersey, I called Jody to tell him how right he'd been, and to wish him a happy birthday. He didn't answer, so I left a message for him to call me as soon as he got back.

On that night, the eve of his birthday, Jody got into Bertha, his big green canoe, and slid onto his beloved river with two friends, Sam and John. Unbeknownst to them, the reservoir gates had been opened upriver. Because of snowmelt, the river was already running unusually high for January. Neither Sam nor John remember exactly how it happened, but not long after they set off downstream, the canoe capsized and the three of them went into the icy black water. They were all dressed in heavy winter clothes, wearing coats and boots. Sam and John abandoned the overturned canoe immediately and swam to shore.

Jody tried to right the canoe and climb back in. Whether it was the shock of cold water that killed him, or the downward suck of his heavy clothes and boots, we'll never know. John thought he remembered Jody shouting he felt as if he was having a heart attack. I couldn't bear to picture him floundering in pain in the water. A paramedic later told me that we fall asleep before we drown, that we aren't aware of the water filling us and pushing us to the bottom. He said that given the temperature that night, it would have been only a matter of minutes before Jody felt nothing. He said that the cold would have slowed his heartbeat, if it was still beating, and he would have felt as if he was going to sleep. There was some solace in picturing Jody falling asleep as he sank to the riverbed.

I got the phone call the next morning as I drove to *POZ* for my second day of work. Melissa, who had married Jody's friend Christian, and who had worked with me at *New Jersey Life*, had the courage to call and tell me what had happened.

It was strange to be on the other side of someone gravely saying, "I have something to tell you."

Somehow, I managed to keep driving into the city and get through my second day at *POZ*, never telling anyone that Jody had died; I didn't yet know the people at *POZ* well enough to cry on their shoulders. And by now, I was practically an expert at handling trauma and mind-numbing sadness by myself.

When I got home, there was a letter waiting for me on the stairs of my barn. Strangely, it was postmarked two years earlier. When I opened it and immediately recognized the familiar handwriting, I sat down hard on the stairs. It was from Jody. Two pages long, it talked about the difficulties we'd had at the end of our relationship, admonishing and, alternately, praising me. But of all the words, several stood out as if they were written in red neon: "If you do nothing else in your life, you must tell the world that you have HIV."

I learned later that Bryce's housekeeper had found the old letter that morning, stuffed in a backlog of mail at his house. We had one mailbox at the farm. They sorted it and when there was a bunch of it, they'd bring it to me. This wasn't the first time a piece of mail had been misplaced. When she found it, she put it on the steps of my barn for me.

Even though news of Jody's death made me feel at first as if I couldn't go on, let alone go back to *POZ* the next day, his words were a divine offering. I knew I couldn't turn my back on the new path he'd helped point out to me. To do so would be to invalidate the memory of all we'd shared. And now that he was gone, that's all I had.

Jody's body remained missing for the next three months. Some days, I imagined he'd faked his own death to escape his small town life and start over somewhere else. Other days, I could feel that he was really gone and I wanted desperately to be out on the river with the boats and helicopters and thick-coated Labradors looking for a sign of him. But despairing as I was, riding up and down the choppy, ice-floe-laden river in vain might have sent me diving into the depths after him. So I pushed my foot down hard on the accelerator and drove like a demon day after day to New York City, trying to work so hard that I had no time, no mental or emotional energy to envision countless iterations of the scene in which Jody sunk below the surface for the last time.

Come spring, I'd settled in at *POZ* and was beginning to get the hang of things. It was refreshing to go to work and talk to people all day long who knew what I was going through. Who could relate and give advice and help educate the world about AIDS. I never had to worry again about going to a doctor's appointment and having my boss or co-workers wonder if there was something really wrong with me.

I was so busy during most of my days that I hardly had time to think about anything other than work while I was at the office. At home, though, things were different. I spent many long, quiet nights missing Jody.

When the weather turned, the thawing river rushed once again, pounding like violent chocolate milk. After months of fruitless hunting, the search team eventually gave up looking for Jody's body. They said if we did find him now, we wouldn't want to see him. But I wanted to see him; to know once and for all if he'd just gone missing or was really gone for good. I ached, thinking of all the stories of people who lost their memory in terrible head injuries. Had he just washed downstream? Was he wandering aimlessly, unsure of where, or who, he was? Or was he really dead?

Pelli, a dear friend of mine who was a therapist, and who'd helped me get back on my feet after my second divorce, called me when she learned the search was called off. She wanted me to know that a psychic working with the state said she had an idea of where Jody lay. Pelli knew that I thought Jody was still in the river and she offered the information as a license to keep looking. She didn't know exactly where he was, only that he was still in the river.

And so, several months after Jody vanished, when the weather turned warm and the water returned to its peaceful sea-bound flow, I started walking the banks every time I could, trying to feel, or sense, whether Jody had really traveled out to sea, or was still in the stretch of river between where they pushed in and where he never came out. I talked to the honking geese that paced along the shore with me. I asked the mallards if they'd seen him.

Back when we first met, I'd introduced him to my hobby of wandering through the woods looking for natural curios, particularly animal bones. He discovered he had a similarly uncanny ability to be drawn toward the one deer carcass in a three-square-acre patch of woods. He called our perception "bone-dar" (like radar), and we spent hours moving slowly through thickets of wild blackberries or oak or cedar forests, or along the riverbank, sometimes on our hands and knees, wearing backpacks, gloves and canvas pants, after a big storm revealed the gifts that nature had left for us.

To search was to be greedy; if we walked the woods needing or expecting to uncover a treasure, it would elude us. But if we moved through nature, open to the hundreds of small ways it spoke to and guided us, we would be drawn to its secret bounty. We both knew the difference between searching—and just being and feeling what was present.

So though I was desperate for an answer, I stopped searching, hoping that his presence would reveal itself to me in time. And then one rainy day, while I was walking along the riverbank under the metal toll bridge that arcs over the river between New Jersey and Pennsylvania, it did. The uneven hammering of the raindrops sounded like a riff Jody used to play on his milky yellow Fender guitar, when we'd sit in his studio above his father's garage on summer nights, writing songs while he tried to persuade me to sing. Listening to the rhythmic drops, I knew he was there with me.

Later, Pelli would tell me that the state psychic, who'd zigzagged from shore to shore hoping to feel Jody as I did, felt his presence in the same spot. So neither of us was surprised when we heard, several weeks later, that a shad fisherman, while placing stakes in the river bottom to guide the competitive shad fishers coming to town for Shad Fest, looked down one late spring afternoon and found Jody lying on the riverbed.

To me, Jody's death seemed an intentional escape on his part; not suicide but a righteous exiting of a modern world whose lack of principles and hypocrisy and technology he never agreed with anyway. The eels had visited his head, taken his eyes, and we weren't allowed to see him. But they told us that his tattoos were still visible: the three black horizontal bars on his shin, the ship's wheel logo on his shoulder—and the fleur-de-lis with "Past Is Prologue" written on his inner forearm.

He was cremated and, afterward, there was a riverside ceremony in the Prallsville Mill, the place we had said our formal good-byes and the site of many a Fire Season concert. Organically, people started going to the front of the room and telling stories about how Jody had inspired them to change who they were before he came into their life. There was a central theme to everyone's story: Jody had pushed us all to be much more than we ever dreamed we could.

I hadn't planned on speaking. I didn't think I could maintain my composure long enough to say anything meaningful. And much of what I felt wasn't appropriate for that audience. But suddenly, I found myself walking slowly to the front of the room. Standing on the stage, I spontaneously told the roomful of strangers, and some friendly faces who had no idea, that I was living with HIV. I told them that because of Jody, I had set aside my fear and shame and taken the job at *POZ*. Come April, I would be open to the world about my HIV status. I managed to get my story out without a single tear.

After we had all told our truth—and how Jody had inspired

us to live it—a smaller group of us set him free again, spreading
his ashes to float in a whitewash along the surface of the river,
which ran beside the mill. One by one, we added a bobbing fleet
of colorful roses. He moved down the Delaware River for a final
time, becoming one again with the forces of nature that he lived
and died by.

After we could no longer see his ashes on the river's surface, I
walked away from the group saying their final good-byes to Jode.
The irony that he'd run from me because he thought I'd die first
hit me in the chest like the kick of a horse. And I fell to my knees
on the sandy riverbank behind a tree and wept a river of tears.

CHAPTER
twelve

Three months later on a sharp March night, I sat curled up in my office at *POZ* feeling incredibly nauseated, clutching my knees to my tumultuous guts. After a decade of doing everything I possibly could to keep my secret, I had followed through on my promise to Jody. I put a photo of myself on *POZ*'s cover above the words: "I am no longer afraid to say I have HIV." I thought that if I said it enough, inscribed it indelibly in a public place, I'd come to believe it. I knew that sharing my story would change everything—but whether it would make anything better for me, or the world at large, was anyone's guess.

Nothing about AIDS circa 2006 was as it should have been. Millions of people around the globe, including children and infants, and tens of thousands of people in America were infected—and dying—every year because people were unable to afford or access life-saving care and treatment. Because of the undiminished stigma, fear and ignorance around HIV, millions of people carried the disease and risked spreading it to others because they were too afraid to get tested for HIV or unaware that they should get tested. We were arguably not much closer to a cure than we were twenty-five years ago when the virus was first identified; and the government, faith-based organizations and the media seemed strangely apathetic. Everywhere, we saw dangerous signs of acute AIDS fatigue. Many of our most brilliant and tenacious AIDS activists were dead, or tired, and I didn't see overwhelming evidence that what was left of the old guard was nurturing future generations of AIDS activists. If more wasn't done, AIDS was going to continue its deadly spread—at a frightening exponential rate.

I didn't know what my disclosure could do for those of us with HIV; I only knew that trying to do something had to be better than sitting back in fear, or complaining. And fighting AIDS publicly gave me an illusion of control in what was certainly a situation that was tragically out of control.

It seemed rational, in the abstract, to remind the world that this disease can happen to anyone. But as I stared at my face on the match print of the cover that was about to go on press the next day, I struggled to believe that this would make a difference. Part of me felt deeply disconnected from the woman I saw staring back at me from POZ's cover. The image of a stern-faced woman in a green V-neck shirt, skinny arms akimbo, hands dug into hips, seemed strangely defiant and tough. The photographer had captured something in my eyes that I had never seen before in my reflection.

Staring and staring at the photo, I finally realized it was resolution—grim resolution that I would stand my ground even if it meant that doing so would be the end of me.

Gripping the shiny replica of the cover that would be printed 150,000 times that night, I went into my creative director's office.

"Can we stop the press?" I asked.

He stared at my end-of-winter pale face, drawn tight with fatigue and anxiety, and he slowly and silently shook his head.

"There's no way, right?"

He just stared at me, shaking his head.

After fifteen years in publishing, I knew the answer but just wanted to hear someone else say it. I leaned against the wall and closed my eyes. My stomach still ached but deep inside something was beginning to let go. There was a strange relief in knowing that my free fall into truth had irrevocably begun. All I really had to do was wait to see what shape I'd be in when I hit the ground.

At 8:40 PM my office phone rang. Who was calling this late? Maybe because the world would soon know anyway, or maybe because I was sick of feeling terribly alone, I answered. Technically, I wasn't supposed to, since for maximum impact we had decided we wouldn't announce my arrival at the magazine until the April issue came out.

The decision to wait until the magazine came out before telling anyone allowed me to get adjusted to working at POZ before being distracted by an onslaught of questions from my friends and extended family, and the world at large; it also gave me the space I needed to deepen my knowledge of HIV/AIDS so that I could speak easily and knowledgeably about all aspects of the pandemic.

I had told my friends, and my former publisher, Cheryl, that I was going to work for a secret start-up and that if it worked out, I could tell them about it come April. I felt awful for having to lie about it, but I believed they would understand, and hopefully forgive me, when I eventually came clean.

Given that it was nearly time to let the beast out of the cage anyway, I lifted the receiver and said, "Hello?"

"Hello, I'm trying to reach the editor of POZ," a woman said.

"Yes, who is this?"

"This is Lia Miller, from the *New York Times*. I'd like to get a quote from the editor for a story I'm writing about AIDS."

Lia. Lia Miller. I'd gone to high school with a girl by that name.

"Lia, by any chance did you go to Princeton Day School?" I asked.

"Yes!"

"Lia," I said slowly, "This is Regan. Regan Hofmann."

"Oh my gosh, how are you?"

"Well, I'm fine, and I'm now the editor of POZ."

"Wow. Why did you take that job?" she asked.

And then, as if someone had given me a shot of truth serum, I said, "I have HIV."

There was a brief silence on the phone.

"How did you get it?" she asked.

"From my boyfriend. Ten years ago."

"Are you okay?"

"Yes," I said.

"That's great," she said. "I mean, great that you're okay."

I told Lia how lucky I was that I'd found out about the infection right away. And that I was still alive because I'd had the support of my family, and money for health insurance and medicine. I told her that I'd come to POZ because I was afraid: afraid that AIDS—a disease that infects more than 56,000 Americans a year—was being portrayed by the media in the United States as "under control"; afraid that women, people of color, young people and people over the age of fifty didn't know they were at significant risk for contracting HIV; afraid that the stigma was worsening; afraid because people still die of AIDS in America— more than 14,000 of them in 2007.

I told her that AIDS has become the number one killer of African American women between the ages of twenty-five and thirty-four. That Latinos represent 18 percent of all new infections. That 50 percent of all new HIV infections in the United States occur in people under the age of twenty-five.

"Lia, you may know this stuff already, but since it seems to never appear in stories about AIDS, I want you to make sure your readers know that this is not a disease confined to gays, blacks, Latinos, poor people, homeless people, drug users, promiscuous people or sex workers. That it is not a gay man's disease any more than it is a disease of white, straight, middle-class women. It's everyone's disease. It's an equal opportunity offender. Infector. Oblivious to behavior, geography, race, ethnicity, gender, age, sex habits, bank balances or morality. A resilient and deadly disease."

There was a long silence after I stopped. I pictured her face, her lips pressed together to keep her jaw from hanging open. Maybe her face was contorted, maybe she was mouthing "oh my gods" and "no ways" to the editor sitting next to her as I unraveled my story. Or maybe she didn't care. I hadn't even considered that horrifying thought.

Then she said, "I was going to ask you for a quote for another story we were thinking about doing on AIDS, but now I think I'd like to write your story instead."

"When would it come out?" I asked.

She cleared her throat. "Monday morning."

It was Friday. That left me roughly sixty hours to tell everyone that I had HIV. Even though the magazine was scheduled to be on the street the next week, I figured I'd have plenty of time to tell the people I knew. *POZ* is distributed at doctors' offices and AIDS service organizations; no one I knew would casually encounter the magazine. But the *New York Times*! Jesus.

"Okay," I said, surprising myself and feeling as if I'd jumped out of a plane without checking to see if I was wearing my parachute.

"Okay! I'm going to tell my editor and we'll call you back," she said, and added, "thank you."

I hung up the phone and looked again at my face on the match print of the cover of *POZ*. I wanted to run for my life. Wanted to sprint to my parking garage, get into my Ford Mustang, drive halfway across the country to our printing press and throw a wrench—literally—into the whole damn thing. Why had I decided to do this?

But it was too late to think about that. Lia called back in a matter of minutes and we got the facts straight. I walked her through the details and avoided answering questions about things I wasn't ready to talk about yet. She told me that the story—along with a reproduction of POZ's cover—would appear in Monday's early edition. She thanked me again and said I was brave. I said that I hoped the article would help someone, somewhere.

I left my office and walked slowly through the empty streets of midtown Manhattan to my parking garage. It was the first of what would be many late nights of walking through Times Square, amazed at how life goes on even as it seems your own life is falling apart. People from all over the world paraded along the streets with faces turned skyward to watch the digital rainbows of color pulsing many stories above them. Though the wind seemed especially cold to me, bare legs flashed and skirts flipped up breezily as passersby laughed and looked up at the five-story-high image of the faces of ordinary people broadcast on the *Time* magazine billboard. Whoever conceived of that billboard was a genius: putting a steady stream of ordinary people on a digital version of the cover of *Time*'s "Person of the Year" issue tapped perfectly into the irrational belief that so many have in New York City: the belief that anything is possible. I saw again in my head the image of myself on POZ's cover and tried not to think about what the exposure was going to mean for me and my family.

As I waited for my car to be retrieved from the garage, I remembered a wintry night many years ago when my parents brought Tracy and me in to see a Broadway play and to have dinner just before the holidays. Tracy and I wore matching felt Crusher hats, Fair Isle sweater sets and pleated skirts. The ruggedness of our wool tights was offset by the polish of our new, matching patent leather shoes. We met some family friends, the Reeds, and their children at an Italian restaurant with an open kitchen in the center. We didn't have to be told to use our best manners. My parents were still in love then, and I watched them look at each other happily as Tracy and I carefully curled our spaghetti on our forks. We remembered to fold our napkins and place them on the table when we asked to be excused to watch the chefs in the glass-encased kitchen crank pasta through shiny silver presses.

"It looks like the Fuzzy Pumper Barber and Beauty Shop," my sister observed, referring to our favorite Play-Doh toy that pushed colorful dough through the perforated heads of dolls so you could shear it off with plastic knives. My sister took my hand absently, as she often did, while we watched the men in white double-breasted suits sculpt pasta. Her habit was an evolution of her thumb sucking; I had become her new safety blanket and even at nine years old, it felt good to be needed. I hung my arm over her tiny shoulders as she stood riveted by the sight of long lengths of fettuccine being draped like fine fabric over brass rods to dry.

We went back to the table and had a full round of desserts. My father, in good spirits further buoyed by martinis, regaled the table with hilarious story after story.

Eventually, my dad and Mr. Reed paid the bill, and we all spilled onto the sidewalk. It had started to snow. I felt as if we were in a freshly shaken snow globe.

Thinking about our family then, it seemed impossible that something as horrific as AIDS would creep into our lives. Now, looking at the wind-reddened cheeks of the kids agape at the city flashing around them, I hoped that they would live their whole lives without knowing the pain that sawed at my gut; the pain of ushering chaos into an otherwise charmed existence.

I got into my car and soon I had driven through the Lincoln Tunnel and out onto the New Jersey Turnpike. The road was blissfully traffic free. It was late at night. I thought about calling my family and telling them about the *Times* piece, but I was too afraid to let them know that the blow would come sooner, and perhaps harder, than we'd imagined. I decided instead to let them sleep and considered how I could orchestrate, over the next few days, a fair disclosure to all those from whom I'd hidden my HIV status for a decade.

While driving down the dark highway the night before my cover was blown by—well, by the cover—I worked on a list in my head that was a cross between a phone tree and a wedding seating chart. There were so many issues to consider. Who should I tell when? Would the order in which I told friends and acquaintances reflect their relative ranking in my list of priorities? I wondered whether people would be upset with me for not telling them for so long. How could I possibly do this without offending people? There was no etiquette book to consult for such a thing. I worried most about telling the Girls Night Out crew. They were going to feel especially deceived: after all the other deeply personal information I had shared with them over the years, I had kept this big nugget from them. I was also really concerned that my best friends from college, Lyerly, Chase and Edie, all of whom were so connected to me that they'd sensed something was awry and asked time and time again throughout the ten-year span if I was "really okay." I'd had so many chances to come clean but I hadn't. Would they ever forgive me?

I dialed Edie in San Francisco, thinking she might still be awake. She might, I thought, be a good first one to tell. But the phone just rang and rang. When it went to voicemail, I remembered it was Friday night. No one I knew was going to be home.

I spoke briefly to my mother on Sunday night—the night before the issue of the *New York Times* with my confession in it hit doorsteps and front porches all over the country. I wanted to tell her but did not know how to express how sorry I was to have to put her through what we both silently feared would be public humiliation on a massive scale. She'd had so much grief already. Frank had died the summer before from bone marrow cancer, and she'd recently lost her beloved Jack Russell terrier, Maggie.

Frank had been diagnosed last July, just prior to my first year at *POZ*, and just after Jody and I broke up. Within a matter of weeks, he was admitted to intensive care. My mom, Tracy and I spent the summer trying to guide Frank through his terrible disease and to handle the shock and sadness of seeing our big strong friend topple and wither. At first, I'd been terrified to visit him at the hospital. I was scared that my slightly weakened immune system would catch some weird superbug. Ever since my diagnosis, I had avoided hospitals like the plague. While a good dose of dirt and bacteria is necessary to keep your immune system on its toes, I didn't want to test whether or not mine could handle the serious stuff.

I was also worried about how watching Frank's demise would make me feel about my own illness. And, of course, I was horrified for Frank and my mom. To be in as much pain as Frank endured and to have to watch someone you love experience that pain are unthinkable things until you find yourself in the midst of them. So I got over my own fears and went to the hospital for Frank, and for my mom.

My mother was extraordinary. She made impossible decision

after impossible decision for Frank's benefit, all the while staying strong and taking care of herself. None of us was relieved when he finally passed away on the day we brought him home to start hospice care. Except maybe Frank.

When my mom called and told me Frank was gone, I drove over to her house, where she was sobbing. With the help of the hospice nurse, I gently got her from the spare bedroom, where Frank lay, to her bed. I covered her with a blanket and asked the hospice nurse what I was supposed to do next.

"Call the undertaker," she said simply.

I sat with my mom until they arrived and then told her to rest while I took care of things.

The two men who had come to collect Frank were his friends; they'd all played golf together. They were also undertakers. I showed them to the room and watched, as they wrapped Frank in a white sheet, carefully and artfully binding it to his body with a silken cord. As I watched, I realized that Frank was not there. The body he had lived in was; but he was already free.

They placed him on a gurney and carried him out the back door and up the hill across the backyard, to the hearse waiting in the driveway.

As we closed the door of the hearse, I realized how much Frank had taught me about life—including how to die with strength and dignity. The greatest gift he gave to me, aside from encouraging me to find the courage to live my life openly with HIV, was to help me through my fear of physical death, convincing me that while the physical body will get disease and eventually disappear, what's inside lives forever.

My mom had done an amazing job coping with her emotions and life in the aftermath of Frank's passing. She was just getting over the shock, and truly the last thing she needed was an assault on her privacy and the pity or disdain of others as a result of my public disclosure. But even if the news struck people the wrong way, I hoped that after the dust settled, she'd find comfort in the aftermath. Maybe this whole thing would help both of us determine who our real friends were. And free us both once and for all from a life bound by secrecy.

I understood that she was afraid for us both, but amazingly she gave me her support, as she always had.

"It's going to be fine. You're doing the right thing," she said. Neither of us entirely believed that, but neither of us challenged it, either.

I said, "I hope so, Mom. I'm really sorry to put you through this."

She didn't respond to that, but only said, "Well, we'll talk in the morning, then. Try to get some sleep."

"Okay. Call me when you see the story."

Next I called Tracy, who said that she was proud of me. "You're going to change the way people think about AIDS—for the better," she said. I marveled at her incredible ability to always cut perfectly to the chase, never failing to give me exactly what I needed to survive. My dad said, simply, "You will help people. It doesn't matter what else happens as long as you're doing that. Call me tomorrow. I love you."

As I lay in bed that last night of my secret life, I wondered whether sharing bad news like this was actually selfish. Maybe if I were tougher, I'd have had the strength to handle this myself. Then I could have spared people the pain of worrying whether I'd get sick and die, spared them the humiliation of having to admit that their daughter/friend/cousin/niece/aunt/coworker/neighbor/sister/girlfriend/ex-wife had HIV.

But also realized I had a right to tell people. After all, I was sick. Didn't I deserve the same help and compassion that anyone who'd been diagnosed with a terminal illness deserved? Still, it was easy to picture the next day going down badly. I imagined an angry throng of neighbors clamoring across the polo field, come to build and burn an effigy of the local girl with AIDS. I wondered whether they'd ban me from the Amwell Valley Trail Association. Would I get the hairy eyeball at the local coffee and pizza places?

I lay awake all night worrying that everyone in my life would think the worst of me. I knew all too well the powerful brew of hysteria mixed for more than twenty-five years around AIDS. Few words had the power to conjure the levels of discomfort and terror you can invoke by saying "AIDS." Not even words like "witch" or "plague" have similar power. I get it, the crazy fear around AIDS. The ingredients mixed in the AIDS brew are particularly potent in their own right: blood, sex, drugs, promiscuity, prostitution, needles, condoms, homosexuality and death.

Sex, in a way, is the central and most troublesome ingredient. Because HIV is sexually transmitted and present in semen and vaginal fluid as well as blood, it forces people to think and talk frankly about sex.

Thinking about getting something deadly from sex makes people have to think about responsibility, culpability. It is the preventable nature of HIV that makes some people believe they have the right to scorn those who have it. Yet what so many people forget, or don't know, is this: it's not that some people have good, clean sex and others have filthy, bad sex; any sex between any two people in any circumstances can allow the virus to pass between them.

The virus doesn't have a conscience. It doesn't gravitate toward any one type of person, one race, one gender, one age group, one sexual orientation or one set of morals or behavior over another. The likelihood of the presence of HIV is simply unpredictable when any two people of unknown HIV status have sex. It is true that certain circumstances make the transmission of HIV more or less possible (the virus dies in the air, it survives in a needle) but the randomness of when HIV is passed along is just that—random.

The connection that people like to make between promiscuity and HIV is misleading, and is really just an excuse for people to erroneously convince themselves that they are not at risk for getting it. While having more sex with more partners certainly increases your chances of getting HIV, your odds of getting HIV are not necessarily low because you have one act of unprotected sex with someone whose status you don't know. We easily believe that a woman can get pregnant from one act of unprotected sex, so why is it so hard to believe that HIV could pass between people as easily as sperm?

The deep irony is that the stigma created by people's unreasonable fear of AIDS—and their intense desire to judge those living with the virus and separate themselves from HIV-positive people by believing that there's a great difference between themselves and positive people—puts them at greater risk for contracting HIV. That's because stigma makes those living with the virus less likely to know their status, treat the disease (treatment can make them less contagious) and disclose.

It's not the decisions or sexual acts that separate people who live with HIV from those who don't. It's just that when we made the same choices as many others do, the retrovirus was present.

Which was why I was doing all this: to show people how very wrong—and potentially deadly—this thinking is.

CHAPTER
thirteen

The Monday that the *New York Times* story appeared, dawn broke over the far edge of the polo field like a submarine, slowly surfacing. The arc of light cast a surreal glow. Red-tailed hawks hunting above the fields curved deliberately around the sky, hooked beaks pointed down as they searched for breakfast. Deer walked on legs like twigs toward the deep grass at the edge of the woods to fall asleep in the spreading sunlight. The horses climbed to the highest point in the pasture to be warmed by the rising sun. No one was in a hurry—but me.

I got up and got dressed in running clothes even though I don't run. You had to have a special arrangement with Shari, my friend who owns Peacock's, the coffee shop down the road, to get a copy of the *Times*, but I didn't want to face her right off the bat, in case she'd seen the story before I had a chance to read it. My neighbors were *Times* subscribers. My plan was to jog over to the end of their driveway, slip their newspaper out of its plastic shield, read the story, fold up the paper, shove it back into the plastic and be on my way before anyone was the wiser. But as I ran down length of our driveway and saw the *Times* lying at the end of the neighbors' driveway, I couldn't bring myself to pick it up.

I couldn't bear to see my story in print quite yet.

Breathing in the icy spring wind and feeling defeated, I meandered back to my house empty handed. My feet crunched down the gravel. If Bryce was awake, he'd see me and wonder what I was doing running past his house at 5:30 AM. Then I remembered that he was on vacation. I imagined him unfurling the *Times* at the ski lodge in Vail and reading about me. I wondered whether he'd call and demand that I leave. I decided that as soon as I got back to the house, I'd pack a bag of my most precious things in case he kicked me out when he got home.

It was too early to call my dad and sister, who now both lived in Santa Fe. My dad had always fantasized about retiring and painting in the high desert. My sister and Josh had moved there shortly after they got married in 2001 to be closer to his family.

By the time I got back to my house, I was wet with sweat despite the March wind. Shaking with a chill and exhaustion from several sleepless nights, I dialed my mother's number. She answered and then said in a soft, firm voice, "The story is good." We didn't say much else and I told her I'd call her later. I knew without asking that she'd been up all night, as I had. I pictured her having her tea and once again felt the familiar wave of guilt caused by putting her through this. But I knew that the parts of me steeled for disclosure came in part from her. The same mettle that propelled me now would allow her to paint a smile on her lips and turn up the morning Elvis show on the radio and brace herself, as I was doing, for the incredulous calls we would no doubt field later that day.

In an effort to delay the inevitable, I showered until there was no more hot water. Stepping out of the tub, I bent at the waist and tossed my hair over my head, rubbing it hard with a towel. I flipped it over my shoulders; it landed with a smack on my back. I stared at myself in the mirror.

I looked surprisingly calm. I tried on a smile. It felt nice. I allowed myself a little congratulatory laugh. I shook my shoulders. The normally steel-like cords that connected my arms to the base of my neck were now soft. Something was different: the dark shadow that had lurked behind my eyes for a decade was gone. It was the fear.

I looked tired, but also younger and happier than I had in a very, very long time. I remembered the meltdown I had had in another bathroom ten years before. Seeing myself in the mirror now, it was hard to believe I was the same person. I was thinner, and older, and the medicines had removed some of the subcutaneous fat from my face, but the loss of my curves was a small price to pay for my life. I was still worried about what would happen that day, but there was some triumph in the mere fact of being here to find out. I didn't think then that I'd still be alive, but ten years later, I was still here, in the flesh.

I dressed and got into my car. I drove out of the driveway, past the hawks sleeping in the sunny treetops, past the horses and past my neighbor's paper—which was lying a little less ominously now in its plastic wrapper at the end of their driveway.

In New York, I parked my car and took the long route to work across sun-soaked Forty-second Street. I checked my cell phone voicemail as I walked; it was full. I listened to encouraging, supportive, lovely messages from people I knew well, and some I barely knew at all. I was overcome; I felt as if I'd been released from death row.

My phone continued to ring all day. More than once, I laughed nervously at the miracle of being instantly freed from fear of rejection by the reconnection with so many people I had cared about over the years. Calls came in to my father, mother and sister; I wondered if they felt the same magnitude of relief at being released from a decade of secrecy and shame.

Somehow, the news spread so far and so fast that people I had even forgotten about contacted me via e-mail, a phone call or a letter.

The most troubling phone calls were from friends whose feelings were hurt, as I'd predicted, because I hadn't told them sooner. Some felt that I didn't trust them to keep my secret safe. Others felt that I'd mistakenly believed they would not have been understanding or compassionate. I tried to explain that I didn't want to burden them with either a secret or worry, and that I had always intended to tell them if I'd gotten sick and needed their help. I told them too that it did me a world of good to be treated as if there was nothing wrong with me. I liked visualizing that I was healthy. And I think doing that helped me stay that way.

I especially worried about my friends with children. If they didn't know any better, they might have been afraid that I'd give HIV to their kids. I remembered a night spent at Lyerly's house. She had made me the co-godmother, along with Chase, of her second daughter, Daphne. From the minute I laid eyes on Daphne, we've been kindred spirits. And though we haven't spent too much time together, when we do, we're pretty much inseparable. One night I stayed over at Lyerly's and woke up eye-to-eye with Daphne's giant baby blues.

She'd climbed into bed with me and I'd slept a few more hours with her folded into my arms.

I had many of these kinds of moments with different friends' children, taking a bite of their cupcake, swimming with them in my arms. As they read the *Times*, would they worry that I'd exposed their kids to AIDS?

When Lyerly first called, and ever since, she'd never mentioned whether she was worried because I'd cuddled with Daphne. I finally brought it up with her, not long ago. She scoffed at me and said, "You can't get AIDS that way!" And I laughed. She was right.

Despite the elation, I remained braced for attacks. I thought: maybe the good news came first. Everyone who wanted to condemn me would call later.

It was true. People who felt fear, disgust, disappointment or disdain didn't bother to write a note and pop it in the mail. They called only when they could no longer suppress their fears or anger or wonderment. Over the six months following my public disclosure, my phone at *POZ* would occasionally ring, and I'd have to withstand a call from a man I dated years before I contracted HIV, wondering whether I had infected him. Amazingly, in many cases it was months between the time these men had heard the news, and when they found the courage to call. In the meantime, they had not gone to get tested for HIV.

In all cases, nothing had ever happened that put them at risk for getting the disease—a fact they understood after we talked.

I walked out of *POZ*'s office after that first day of my disclosure, and stopped into Sephora to buy myself a new shade of bright lipstick. I wanted the whole world to see my smile, now that I was anonymous no more.

CHAPTER
fourteen

I have read *Vogue* since I was a little girl shuffling around the house in a pair of my mother's too-big patent leather sling-backs, pretending that I was going to a fancy party. From the age of nine, I have eagerly awaited the magazine's appearance in my mail-box. It showed up like an eccentric, overdressed relative from the city—totally out of place among the weeds and wildflowers of our farm, but welcome nonetheless. The fantastical pictures of the razor-thin women with painted faces, adorned in clothes and diamonds with pheasant feathers in their hair, the metallic type and deeply saturated color of its pages, and the sheer heft of its shiny glamour were powerful antidotes to my sequestered, sepia-toned rural life spent mucking horse stalls and endlessly removing, according to the season, the leaves, the sticks and the snow from the driveway.

As a little girl, I would tape the glossy pages of *Vogue* to the walls of my bedroom in our farmhouse, making floor-to-ceiling glitzy collages of fashion. It seemed absurd for a girl who spent her life in jeans and rubber boots to worship at the altar of couture, but even back then, I dreamed that one day, my life would take a twist so that I would have places to wear one-shouldered gowns or boots so shiny they looked wet. I liked imagining I'd have an occasion to don a dress covered in a swath of pale gray emu feathers cascading from my throat down to platinum-beaded sandals. With maybe a top hat. My love affair with *Vogue* was one of the reasons I wanted to work at a magazine—and why I eventually started, wrote for, and edited several of them.

I always fantasized about being on the cover of a magazine, in the same unrealistic way that young girls imagine themselves as leading ladies, or princesses. Never in a million years though did I imagine I'd actually be on one—especially on the cover of a magazine about AIDS.

After the article about me ran in the *New York Times*, an editor at *Vogue* asked if I would like to write about having HIV for their June issue.

Midnight the night before my article was due, I paced around my barn, alternately beating myself up for leaving the writing of the piece until the eleventh hour and knowing that without the gun-to-the-head pressure of a deadline hours away, I wouldn't have written a word.

Though I'd been a writer all of my professional life, it was much harder than I thought to describe what it was like to live with HIV—even after I'd taken the initial plunge of public disclosure. It was agonizing to try to render emotions I'd kept locked away for a decade. To do so, I had to go back in time to the most painful moments of my life. But after spending hours circling my laptop, which was perched on a tiny table behind a brown velvet love seat looking out the glass doors of the second story of my barn, I finally sat down and hammered the piece out. I wrote without a thought about what the women who read *Vogue* would think of me and my repulsive, terribly unfashionable disease. If

I managed to tell my story right, maybe more women would be-lieve this could happen to them and not end up like me.

Reducing a decade of fear, denial and depression (and brief moments of overcoming those things) into a 1,500 word story about AIDS served up for mainstream consumption seemed impossible. How could I summarize the arc of my journey from abject fear to realizing that most days I didn't even think about AIDS until it was time to take my pills at night? And, perhaps most important, how could I reassure people they had nothing to fear from those of us living with HIV while simultaneously scar-ing them sufficiently so that they would change their behavior, take precautions and avoid getting it?

In between stints of writing—the paragraphs came quick and hot as if forced through the nose of a shotgun—I paced around the barn.

I had desperately wanted to write this piece and now that I had to, I desperately wished I'd never been asked to do it.

To further procrastinate, I decided to go online and look up *Vogue*'s circulation. It was 1.2 million: one point two million women, girls, teens, tweens, grandmoms, fashionistas, editrixes, soccer moms who love Hedi Slimane, women in their seventies who can still rock Dior, women in their twenties who can af-ford Balenciaga, women who can spell, properly pronounce, pay for and pick out of a crowd the two men comprising Proenza Schouler. One point two million women who would soon know that HIV could happen to them, too.

I was embarrassed to admit that I'd been stupid enough to have unprotected sex without getting tested with my partner first. But if I did, maybe other women wouldn't find themselves in the same situation. One point two million was a lot of lives. It was also a lot of people who could say that I was a tramp, a fool, an idiot, an inconsequential waste of a woman. But if my story could save their lives, I really didn't care what they said about me.

When I grew tired of pacing, I poked at the computer keys with my eyes closed slightly so I couldn't see the words too clearly. My life story looked different on the screen. The letters of the alphabet were comfortingly familiar, but the words, phrases and sentences gave an uncomfortable permanence to what had existed mostly as a bad dream I tried to shake off during my waking hours. Writing it down in greater detail than ever before, the full horror of my story became real to me in a way I had never previously allowed.

Finally, night quieted the barn. The cats tired of creeping around and hunting every suggestion of movement. Everything was still. The pink light of the sun hovered beneath the lip of the darkness, allowing the night creatures to settle in before the flaming star of the sun unveiled tomorrow. The owls moved to their daytime perches in the upper branches of the cedar trees, softly hooting, and the horses made their way to the crest of the small hill in the pasture to be ready to catch the first warmth of the new day. My story was done. I decided to send it without rereading it. Otherwise, I would never let it go.

I did it: the details of ten years of silence around HIV were recorded for the first time in digital, invisible molecules of frightening truth and were sent flying through the last of the night from satellite to satellite. Sometime the next day, *Vogue*'s editor, Ms. Wintour, would read and share it with 1.2 million women. Women who would otherwise, as I did once, perceive themselves to be immune to a virus that knows no bounds, despite our attempts to assign it only to the disenfranchised, the promiscuous, the derelict, the dirty and the bad.

I decided to make it clear that I got HIV from unprotected sex, because one of the first questions people asked me was always, "How did you get it?" As if that has any bearing on what is vital. I wish people would ask instead: how I will survive, if I will survive, if the rest of my life will be worth living, if I will be brave and strong enough to face what might come.

I can't imagine someone telling me they have walking pneumonia and my asking, "Well, now, how did you get *that?*" The "how" with AIDS is so important because it is the thing that people use to barricade themselves from the fear produced by my disclosure. The faster they can separate themselves from me, the quicker they can stop worrying that the disease will—or might have already—infected them, too. If they can ascertain that I was a wanton woman with a propensity for massive amounts of sex, they can put me in an entirely different category. If only they can hear that I shared filthy needles with whores while shooting heroin in a drug den, or if perhaps I had an organ transplant in rural China and was given tainted blood products, then they can rest easy that AIDS will not enter their bodies and ruin their lives. But the truth—that I got HIV from two times of unprotected sex with a straight man—makes them more uncomfortable than it does me when I say it. That is the point. We must all face our discomfort about speaking frankly about sex to stop other people from dying. It is too late for me; it is not too late for others.

Five days passed after I sent the article. The agonizing wait to see what would come of it reminded me of days spent awaiting lab results. Every three months when you have HIV they prick your vein and draw syringe after syringe of burgundy blood into glass vials, releasing the thick rubber tubing from around your bicep only after the eighth or ninth vial when it seems that there can't possibly be much more blood left in you.

I learned to like certain parts of the lab test ritual—like the clicking together of the blood-filled tubes that sounds like thin frozen sticks rubbing together in an ice storm. Sometimes I got a Princess Bride Band-Aid, or maybe a Hello Kitty one, to hide the small wound on the inside of my elbow. I always felt cleaner after they sucked out so much of my infected blood.

Before I got my latest blood work results back, the answer came from *Vogue*. They liked the piece and agreed to run the article.

Days after it was accepted, *Vogue*'s fact checker called to confirm the details of my story. All was going smoothly until she asked for the name and contact information for the man who had given me HIV.

"I can't give that to you," I said.

"We're going to need that for the piece," she insisted.

"I'm sorry, but I just can't."

She got testy with me, explaining the importance of accuracy in journalism and asking that I, especially as a journalist, help her do her job.

"I just can't give it to you," I said one more time.

"Why not?" she said, exasperated.

"Because he's dead," I finally said.

"Oh my god, I'm sorry," she said.

So was I.

I'd heard that Antonio had passed away the year before I took the job at *POZ*. Jill, a dear friend of mine who knew I'd dated him, called me at work one day. After some small talk she said, "Listen, I wanted to tell you that I heard Antonio died. And someone said he died of AIDS. I thought you'd want to know, you know, in case . . ."

"Oh my god," I said with real shock. When I was last in touch with anyone who knew him, maybe eight years prior, I had heard that he had gotten married and was doing well. We hadn't stayed in touch.

Since I hadn't disclosed, I didn't want to tell Jill that I was carrying a legacy of my time with Antonio. So I did something I hated to do: lie to a close friend. "I've gotten tested for HIV and am okay," I said to her, crossing my fingers and wishing then that it could have been true.

"That's good to hear," she said.

Later, when I finally did come forward, I called her, explained the situation and thanked her for her extreme bravery in calling me to let me know. It couldn't have been easy to do. She said she appreciated it and told me I was going to be okay and asked me to call her if I ever needed help.

And so, when the *Vogue* fact checker pushed me to the point of having to tell her that Antonio was dead, I cried all the tears I never allowed myself when I first heard he'd died. The day Jill tried to help me save my own life.

After work, I really wanted to go to the barn and spend some soothing time with the horses but I knew that many of the other women who kept their horses at the barn probably read *Vogue*, and I just didn't feel like facing their scrutiny.

A week after the issue of *Vogue* containing my story hit the news-stands, I pulled into the barn. It was dusk. A thin lunar slice had appeared on the horizon with the authenticity of a paper moon being hoisted above the set of a high school play. Deer grazed in the fields; the grooms had yet to turn the horses out for the night.

I parked the car and as I was about to get out, I saw the hulking frame of a chestnut mare step behind my car. A woman stepped out of the barn, then another, and two more rode up on horseback. They surrounded the car, waiting for me to get out. My throat constricted and I took a drink of water, stalling.

I finally opened the door and looked at the women dressed in fancy European britches and gleaming black custom-made leather boots. They stared at me. The one I knew best, a pretty, jaunty woman named Lorraine, whose hair was the same ruby red as her horse's hide, started to clap. She beat her gloved hands together slowly in a dull leather thump. The other ladies joined in. I smiled wanly, still not sure why they were there—or why they were clapping.

"You're very brave," Lorraine said.

"We read *Vogue*," another woman said.

"Thank you," I said to both at once.

And they stepped in closer, tossing questions and praise and comfort into our small circle. I couldn't say a word because I was absolutely overcome by their support, and I didn't want to cry when everyone was being so very kind and saying that I was such a strong woman.

I listened to them talk about AIDS, how surprised they were that I had it, and how they planned to call their daughters and speak to them about it, how well I looked, all things considered, and how great it is that you can get HIV and still survive. Standing among them I thought: five women down, 1.2 million more to go.

CHAPTER

fifteen

Part of the happy fallout that occurred as a result of my disclosure was that I reconnected with many friends with whom I'd lost touch over the years. Not surprisingly, many of them had children. Maybe because I was now receiving an onslaught of baby pictures as I caught up with people from my past, or maybe because my fortieth birthday was approaching, I began to focus on the question of motherhood.

I had never caught baby fever. Partly that was because I had yet to meet a man I wanted to have a child with, and partly it was because I'd spent the better part of my adult life feeding, cleaning up after, loving and supporting legions of animals; my nurturing nature had been well-exercised by that point. Ironically, I had lived long enough to possibly be too old to have a healthy child, even though modern medicine made it possible for women to lower their viral load to an undetectable level and have HIV-negative children. That made me sad.

And by that point, my sister and Josh had a beautiful son who was the light of all of our lives, and who, in the few precious weeks I'd spent with him, showed me the difference between loving a horse, a cat and a child—especially one who was related to you.

Seeing how he embodied his parents' physical and other traits rekindled my regret that if I had to leave the planet prematurely, I couldn't leave a part of me behind in a child.

I've always thought the idea of wanting a child in the abstract seemed absurd—and selfish. I imagined I'd meet a man who I loved so much that I'd want more of him, in the form of a child. And whom I adored to the point of wanting to mix my DNA to see what kind of genetic imprint we could make together. But as I was nowhere near that point in my life at the time, I set dreams of a baby aside.

I reminded myself that there were millions of orphaned children around the world—nearly 15 million of them had lost their parents to AIDS. If I really felt the need to raise a child one day, I told myself I'd adopt. Although the authorities might not let an unmarried, HIV-positive woman be an adoptive mom, even to a child that no one else wanted, from time to time I wrote versions of a letter I hoped would overcome any barriers should the day come that I'd be ready and in a position to give a child a new life.

Still, all these solutions, while making me feel better, felt like a consolation prize—a sad second to the real deal: having my own child with a man I loved.

But while all these thoughts had ricocheted around in my head, I had never talked about them out loud. Until, that is, I did so in front of millions of people on live national television. Soon after the *Vogue* article appeared, a producer from *Good Morning America* asked me to appear on the show. My first job out of college was as an intern at CBS News when Diane Sawyer was there, and from the moment I read about her career trajectory from a Junior Miss beauty queen to a network news anchor, I have admired her immensely. I knew she was one of the hosts of GMA and I hoped she would interview me. I was happy but surprised that GMA would do a show about AIDS. I didn't think they went to such serious places that early in the morning.

The thought of appearing on GMA absolutely terrified me. I told the magazine's owner that I wasn't sure I could do it. So he hired a media trainer to ready me for my first national TV exposure. Nellie arrived at *POZ* the next day and we spent nine grueling hours in the conference room under the unforgiving fluorescent lights. She filmed me with a hand-held video camera and played back the tape on a monitor to show me what I would look like on TV.

I looked like a praying mantis. On crack.

I bobbed and weaved; my eyes were the size of Ping-Pong balls. Nellie patiently gave me advice and I tried to apply it. She showed me playback after playback of my attempts to do as she directed; after about an hour, I started to panic because there seemed to be no way I was going to pull it together in time not to embarrass myself publicly. I really didn't want to look like a freak on national television. I could barely stand the image of myself waving my hands spastically in the air end trying to keep a look of upbeat resolve on my face while discussing the devastating impact AIDS had had on my life. And I wondered why I never noticed before how far my ears stick out from my head.

It was painful, but I pushed myself through the agony of seeing my frightened, awkward self on the monitor. I desperately wished I had participated in even one school play. It seemed impossible to go from being the kind of person who could not bear to stand and make a toast at a family birthday to being someone who could be comfortable, articulate and normal-looking on live daytime television—in the span of twenty-four hours.

But with Nellie's expert cajoling, by the end of our time together, I felt I might not make a public disaster of myself. Unless
they asked me highly personal questions and I answered, as Nellie had specifically instructed me not to, without thinking. The
most valuable thing Nellie taught me was how to "bridge"—how
to respond to a question without answering it, redirecting the
conversation to a new topic.

We practiced.

"So, Regan," she said, "what did you think about the man
who infected you when you discovered he was HIV-positive?"

"Well, it's important to remember that protecting yourself is
the responsibility of all people involved in sex, and that what
someone looks like is no indication of whether or not they're
positive."

She smiled. Her work was done.

Nellie told me that the majority of what people think of you
on TV is based on what you look and sound like, not what you
actually say. As long as I sat up straight, smiled, looked calm and
confident, she said I'd make a fine impression.

The next step in my media makeover was meeting with a
woman named Laura, who POZ had hired as my publicist and
who was in charge of shopping with me for an outfit. The first
thing she said was that I needed a killer suit.

"I don't wear suits," I told her. "I wear jeans. Every day."

"Well, you can't wear jeans on *Good Morning America*," she said.

She carted me to a Lower East Side boutique that sold im-
ported designer suits for half off. But despite her attempts to convince me that the right suit would make me feel invincible, it
didn't, especially the St. John and Escada ensembles I tried on
that made me look, respectively, like a first-lady-wannabe and a
sailor. But as I was so new to all this and she was an accomplished
professional, I dutifully stripped down time and time again, stuff-

ing myself into pants and skirts and blazers, parading up and down the cold linoleum floor of the boutique so she and a bevy of middle-aged men who owned the store could give each outfit the thumbs up, or down.

In the end, I came back from the shopping excursion empty handed, save for a bag of homemade pickles from the Jewish deli near the store. I ate the whole bag of pickles in the taxi before realizing that eating that much salt in one sitting was bound to make me look like a blowfish on TV the next day. I guessed it was better to look like a blowfish than a praying mantis.

The morning I was scheduled to appear on GMA, I got out of bed at 4:30. I didn't have to wake up, because I never fell asleep. As I drove due east from the New Jersey countryside into Manhattan, straight into the rising sun, I listened to a CD Lyerly had made for me. It was full of songs of empowerment. Lord knows I needed to steel myself. I swung my Mustang aggressively around the last twists of highway that brought me to the mouth of the Lincoln Tunnel.

It was one thing to tell my story from the privacy of my house and later see it appear on the pages of *Vogue*. It was another thing entirely to tell my story in real time to millions of people who were getting dressed, frying eggs and packing up their kids' books for school. I tried to stay calm, but I kept picturing Diane Sawyer asking me the first question and me just freezing, open mouthed, staring dumbly into the camera.

When I got to the office I was met by a hair stylist and Erin, the second publicist POZ hired to help me. I continued to feel ill as the stylist blew my hair out. I wished she could blow the knots out of my intestines. As I sat in my office at POZ speculating about what the morning would bring, Erin was incredibly encouraging and supportive. She kept telling me there was nothing to worry about. But she was not the one going on TV.

Erin reminded me that three minutes is a very short amount of time.

"You can do anything for three minutes," she said, cheerful as a sparrow.

I thought of a lot of things I didn't think I could do for three minutes. Like lower my face into a vat of boiling water. Or eat a handful of live lizards. Or talk about having HIV on *Good Morning America*. The stylist put a final layer of spray lacquer on my hot-ironed curls and I looked at my reflection in the glass wall of my darkened office. My hair had been curled back in a long flip, rising up from either side of my face. It reminded me of the hair of one of my babysitters when I was growing up. The one who stayed with Tracy and me when we lived in Southern California. Thinking of my babysitter made me think of Tracy. And my parents. Suddenly I was overcome, desperately missing my family.

Erin and I walked from *POZ*'s offices through Times Square to the ABC studio. I felt pretty good—until I looked up and saw the big wavy billboard with live video of GMA flashing across it. I stopped in my tracks just before the entrance to the studio. Erin took a firm grip on my elbow and led me to the door. A security guard inspected his clipboard. As he hunted for my name, I looked at the names of the other guests also scheduled to appear that day. Michael Keaton was coming. I felt much better, knowing Batman would be in the building. After finding my name, the guard urged me inside, where I was greeted by a flurry of people.

After what seemed like a year, they took me out onto the set and asked me to stand on the edge of the beautifully lit studio. Between the makeup and the lighting, at least my skin was going to look amazing. While I waited in the wings, I noticed a group of kids they'd brought up from the street. Every day, they allow tourists to visit the set. One little girl leaned toward another and asked, "What's *she* here for?" pointing at me. The other cupped her hand over her mouth and whispered viciously just loud enough for me to hear, "She's got *AIDS*. I heard them say it when she came in."

I smiled wanly at the kids and tried to remind myself that responses like theirs were the very reasons I was about to possibly humiliate myself in front of tens of millions of Americans unsuspectingly eating their cornflakes.

As a preamble to my segment, GMA rolled footage of the early days of AIDS showing skeletal people wrapped in paper-like skin hooked up to IVs; half-dead babies with flies crawling around their eyes and former President Ronald Reagan, who refused to acknowledge that there was such a thing as AIDS until it was way, way, way too late.

I'm not sure if it was the images and the indecency of what so many people have had to endure while trying to survive AIDS, or the lingering sting of the little girl's words, but I suddenly felt my eyes fill with tears. I tried to smile, straighten my vertebrae and distract myself from the terrifying images that reminded me where my own body might be headed one day. Shoulder blades like hangers; flies on my dead face, the never banishable image of a toe tag . . . these were not good things to see before having to stand strong in front of so many strangers. But before I could even process how upset I was, they escorted me to an armchair beside Diane Sawyer. I felt so scared that my body shut down and within seconds, I was blissfully numb.

I sat primly on the edge of my armchair as Nellie had instructed me to do with my feet flat on the floor and the palms of both hands placed primly on my bent knees. I looked at Diane Sawyer, transfixed by her blue eyes.

"How are you?" she asked.

"I'm good. Thank you for having me on the show," I choked out.

"Look here, at me," she said. "Not directly into the camera.

And don't be nervous. Only millions of people will be watching."
She smiled widely.

Suddenly, without warning, she was talking to America and
I felt like a bug pinned alive to a scientist's examination table.
She fired question after question at me, all the while looking
deeply into my eyes and sending me waves of sympathetic energy. Her questions were pointed but her delivery was laced
with compassion.

How did I get HIV? she wanted to know. Was I mad at the
man who gave it to me? How did my parents react? Did I worry I
was going to die? What was it like to date with HIV?

"Tell me, Regan," she asked, "would you ever consider having
a baby?"

I looked at the little kids standing at the edge of the stage,
trying to gather some strength. They were a touchstone for me.
Maybe if I managed to tell my story compellingly enough, they
wouldn't grow up not knowing about HIV. And I thought about
the POZ staff and the work we did trying to correct all the misperceptions that exist about AIDS. One of the biggies is that
people don't know that HIV-positive women, and men who wash
the HIV from their sperm via with a new technique, can have a
healthy, HIV-negative child. So even though a child of my own
wasn't in my imminent future, I said, "I'd love to have a child,
someday."

"And positive people can do that now?"

"Yes, as long as I am on antiretroviral medicines. If I gave my
baby medicine at and just after birth and didn't breast feed, the
chance that it would be positive is less than two percent."

The three minutes they allocated for my segment came and
went; Diane Sawyer waved off the producer, who indicated that
our time was up. I had a moment of panic. I had only been coached
to handle three minutes. At the end of our chat, which stretched

to an ungodly seven minutes (time does not pass the same way when you're on TV), her eyes welled up and she gripped my arm. I leaned forward and we stayed attached, looking at each other on a set that went silent even though there were about forty people standing around.

Finally, she nodded at me, let go and turned away, moving to the next set while everyone bustled onto the next part of the show. As I walked off set, the kids just stared at me. The little girl who'd had so much disdain in her voice looked at me wide eyed. I wanted to get her name and number and call her one day and ask whether hearing my story had changed what choices she would make about sex, her body and her life.

I went back to the green room, collected my stuff and walked out through the set. The show was still airing. The executive producer passed me as I exited, shaking my hand and saying that I'd done "great." I felt like a balloon that had been inflated with helium but not tied closed. Someone was pinching my neck, holding the gas in, and the minute there was release, I would shoot wildly around the room until there was no air left in me and I'd fall limp, hollow and rubbery to the floor. But I was elated.

I walked back to the *POZ* office. It was only 8:30 AM and there was no one else at the office. I called my mom but her phone was busy. I could only imagine the calls she'd be getting. It was too early to call my dad and Tracy; they would still be sleeping. So I changed into jeans and marveled at the irony of feeling so alone after sharing such intimate news with millions of strangers.

I checked my email. There was a nasty message from a man in the Midwest who was furious that I said I would consider having a baby. "How could you be so selfish?" he wrote. "How could you risk the life of a child just so you could have a baby?" I was stunned by the harshness of his words. I decided to write back to him and set him straight. Rather than be mad, I was gentle in my tone and asked, politely, that he reconsider his stance.

Within twenty minutes, he sent back a lovely, apologetic email. He said he appreciated my taking the time to educate him; he'd no idea that an HIV-positive woman could safely have a child, with minimal risk to the father and baby. (He had also asked how I could get pregnant without infecting my partner. I explained I'd use IVF.) If I could change this man's view of people living with HIV with one email, then my plan for asking the world to be more benevolent toward those with the disease just might work after all.

When I first found out that I was HIV-positive in 1996, they told me that if I became pregnant, the risk to my child would be great; at the time, they estimated that there was nearly a 25 percent chance that I'd pass the virus along to my baby. For years, it was hard to tell whether I really didn't want a child or whether I did, but because I knew I couldn't, I shoved that desire deep down inside of me to a place where it couldn't be summoned out—not even by the sight of adorable towheaded tots smiling at me from strollers.

Letting go of such a basic instinct as wanting to have a child is a very hard thing, and I tried to do it by constantly reminding myself that I had gotten a reprieve from death and should be grateful even if I had to live my life in a more limited way than before.

To overcome my "survival depression" I made a list of things that were good about living a long time: being able to care for my aging parents; sticking around long enough to see my sister become a mother; maybe even living to see the end of AIDS. But never in my wildest fantasies of future happiness did I ever allow myself to put "have a child" on the list of reasons I was glad to be alive.

Even though I eventually came to understand that the risk of transmission was low, I worried about becoming so involved with a man that we'd want to have a baby together, manage to have the baby and then die on them both. Was that fair? Maybe it was. After all, it wasn't any different than when any two people fall in love and have a child hoping for the best.

Between those early days of having to accept all that I would miss by dying early and the years I spent reacclimatizing to what might hopefully prove to be a long life, I realized I did not want a baby in the abstract; I wanted to meet someone with whom I desperately wanted to have a child. I wanted to love someone so much that I would be ready to give up huge chunks of myself, my time, my energy, my body, my dreams, my career, my aspirations, all to impart what is critical for a child to be happy, safe and succeed.

My mother gave up so much for me and my sister, and my father worked so hard to give us every tool we needed to make our way in the world. I wondered whether I had the same strength to offer a child the same kind of life my parents afforded me.

Though today I wish I could have my own child, I have come to accept that it may be my destiny to be the best aunt ever to my sister's children and to all my friends' little ones and maybe, someday, to help children orphaned by AIDS. And maybe even bring one home.

CHAPTER

sixteen

Several months later, the shock and awe of my disclosure was over and I was settling into the routine of the things I did regularly before my life had been turned upside down by media coverage.

Which is how I found myself on the Fourth of July weekend wandering the aisles of the Golden Nugget, the same flea market where my mom and I had found the gypsy funeral wagon years before. I was feeling a little sorry for myself that I'd be spending another holiday alone when I bumped into Dan, a long-haired, artistic man from a neighboring town whom I hadn't seen in about a year but had always had a big crush on.

I was trying on vintage military coats when I felt fingers at the nape of my neck. I turned and saw my reflection in a pair of Ray-Bans. Dan's hand stayed on my neck sending a wave of electricity down my body. I'd told him I was HIV-positive several years prior, when we'd first met, but even if I hadn't, I'm sure he would have heard through the grapevine by then.

I'd gone into his antique store one day looking to add to my collection; I'd seen a jar of blue starfish in the window of his shop one night as I walked past. We chatted that day and several more days, until one late afternoon, our conversation continued into dinner and an unexpected kiss outside of my car one night. I had to stop him before our lips met, so I could tell him I had HIV.

By the time I told Dan, I was getting used to the patterns of disclosure. So when he recoiled visibly, I neither took it personally nor worried that that would be his final response to me. Indeed, he got over the idea of the HIV. He placed his favorite necklace over my head one night, and said he was "working through the HIV." It was a strangely tender gesture. He couldn't touch me but wanted me to wear something that made me think of him every second of every day, while he mulled over whether or not he could come to terms with my disease. It felt like an emotional place holder.

But several weeks later, he confessed that he'd opted for another woman with the excuse she could cook, worked many fewer hours and fit his bill of wanting to find someone to "take care of him." I suspected it wasn't true. He was afraid of the "high-five," as I'd taken to calling HIV.

That day at the flea market, several years later, as his touch lingered on my nape, I felt that he might finally have worked through the HIV. So with the hot sun cooking me in the vintage heavy wool soldier's coat, I smiled invitingly at him.

"I like the navy one," he said. "Try it on again."

I slid out of the itchy coat and he helped me into a double-breasted pea coat, brushing the backs of his knuckles across my throat while fastening the toggles.

"Want to go see the fireworks?" he asked.

He looked like a cleaner version of Johnny Depp in *Pirates of the Caribbean*.

"Sure," I said as coolly as I could.

"I'll call you later," he said. And with that, he flashed me a smile and walked away.

Later, I found myself wondering whether he would call.

HIV kept me on my toes. Just as diabetics often become healthier post-diagnosis, I think my fear of rejection because of HIV has pushed me to be a better woman in every way I can think of. I want no one to have any other excuse to reject me and so I try really hard to improve all parts of me that are changeable. But as the hours passed without a call from Dan the feeling I dread most started to well in me. I couldn't derail the thought that if only I was_____(fill in the blank) I would be good enough for a given guy despite the HIV.

While I waited, twisting the situation around in my mind, I painted my toenails.

Finally, Dan called and said he was having a party at his house. And fireworks. And just like that, my fear disappeared.

I was feeling pretty good when I arrived at his house. I parked my car, walked through a large crowd of people spilling from the kitchen out onto the terrace and saw Dan. While we were smiling at each other through the throng, my horses' acupuncturist, James, who'd last seen me several years ago when my hair was short and dark, spied me. Waving vigorously, he boomed across the crowded party for all to hear, "Well, look at you! Long blond hair and AIDS and all!"

The whole party fell silent and stared at me.

Go on, I said to myself, lift the corners of your mouth and smile. Let the smile slide all the way up to your eyes and engulf your whole face. Show them it's okay. That you are not afraid. That there is no shame in having HIV. Walk up to Dan despite the fact that he's staring at you, stricken, and kiss him on the cheek and say hi in a sexy voice. Be brave. Smile.

But before I could manage insouciance, the people at the

party tired of waiting for me to snap out of my frozen, awkward surprise and they turned back to each other. The conversation started rumbling again. Dan turned his back to me and kept cooking at the stove.

A voice at my elbow said, "Do you need a drink?"

It was Oliver, my cats' vet.

"Please, that would be great. Wine. White, please," I stammered. "A big glass."

James came over and said he preferred me as a blonde. When he'd seen me last my hair had been jet black and hacked off at my jaw line. We met when I called him to help me try to save Lucy, a very sick polo pony that a friend had given me to rescue.

James had diagnosed Lucy when the regular vets could not. He had run his hands all over her body and poked and prodded her and eventually told me her liver was shot. He recommended that I take her to the local clinic to get an ultrasound of her abdomen; he was right. It turned out she'd eaten a poisonous plant before I got her and the effects were irreversible. He helped me by giving me the information I needed to make the decision to end her suffering. He was an amazing man and though he'd embarrassed me at the party, he wasn't being intentionally unkind.

I couldn't hold a grudge against him because of his greeting; I did look shockingly different than the day he told me I had to put Lucy down. And in a way, his response was what I was hoping for from the whole world—to treat HIV like any other thing someone might casually refer to at a party.

Toward the end of the party, Dan, who recovered when he saw others were okay with my HIV, and I eventually got some time to hang out alone. Seeing that I was not a social pariah—people had still circled around me and talked and laughed with me all night even after hearing I had HIV—he allowed himself to publicly acknowledge that we were together by laying his hand on my knee.

One of his hobbies was to make videos, pairing footage of everything from eighth-grade science films, to burlesque dancers, to tiny fawns grazing, with music that had nothing to do with the images. He showed the films on the side of his house and I sat curled under his arm around a fire pit for hours watching his creations. He dragged his finger slowly up my bare forearm, when he thought others weren't looking.

As it got later, and guests got sparser, I wondered how he would handle the tension that was building between us. I wondered whether the HIV would unplug the electrical flow that I felt in his fingers.

The sky split open with light and rumbled and growled as we finished the last of the wine at his dining room table while the storm thundered on the roof.

Eventually, he kissed me tentatively and then we talked some more. Well after midnight, the rain stopped and we went outside to sit by the smoldering fire. From the courtyard I could see through glass windows into a studio opposite the house. A cast iron bed with rumpled sheets sat in front of a wood-burning stove. He watched me check out his lair and though his eyes indicated that some part of him considered taking me there, he touched my face tenderly and said, "It's late. You must be tired."

I left, but for the first time, driving away from what was certainly a kind and gentle rejection, I felt fine. Relieved even.

As I wound along deserted back country roads, I told myself that even though HIV hampered my sexual freedom in one sense, it provided invaluable insight that freed me in another it kept me from ending up with people who were wrong for me. When I told people that I had HIV, I could see from their first reaction what their intention toward me might be. And though part of me wanted him to invite me to lie in the fireside bed with him, I did not want to be with anyone who was uncomfortable with HIV, which he clearly was.

Had the circumstances not included HIV, I would have been put off if Dan had invited me into his bedroom on the first night. I realized that if I took HIV out of the equation and considered how Dan had treated me, he had not been nearly gracious enough, nor had he done enough wooing to warrant having the pleasure of my intimate company, long blond hair, AIDS and all.

CHAPTER

seventeen

A month later, as part of my responsibilities as *POZ*'s editor, I was sent to the International AIDS Conference (IAC). Held that year in Toronto, the conference is like the Super Bowl of AIDS—bringing together some of the world's best researchers, scientists, activists, pharmaceutical executives, governmental leaders, artists, journalists, radical thinkers, alternative healers and others who care about stopping the epidemic.

Gathering more than 26,000 people from all over the world, the International AIDS Conference is an amazing spectacle of humanity. On the one hand, the conference is formal: the schedule of sessions and press conferences is tight, security and media clearance are necessary and many of the scientists, researchers and pharmaceutical executives wear suits. World leaders, celebrities and famous figures of the AIDS world speak, and their remarks are fed by satellite all over the world. On the other hand, the conference is primal: tribal leaders dance around the Global Village in grass skirts and porcupine quill crowns, Masai Mara women sell beads to pay for their AIDS medications and Brazilian fashion designers display evening gowns made from hundreds of colored condoms. There are salons, workshops, guerrilla video crews, demonstrations and secret meetings of the community underground.

I was in awe of the spectacle around me.

People flowed up and down escalators, moving to and from plenary sessions, lectures, panels, workshops—and in the Global Village, people from all over the world gathered to swap stories of survival.

In between presentations and meetings, I rushed back to the media center to post or edit stories on poz.com and to attend press conferences.

One day, while walking to get a Diet Coke, I saw a familiar face: that of my AIDS doctor, Dr. Wilson, a kind-eyed, tall, fit man with a swish of sandy brown hair. Though he lived near my hometown and I occasionally saw him while shopping or having dinner at a local restaurant, we had never before acknowledged each other in public. He was protecting my privacy and, before I disclosed, I was terrified that even nodding to him would out my HIV status to the world. It was always awkward bumping into Dr. Wilson in public and having to pretend I didn't know him. He'd seen me virtually naked. He had helped save my life. And yet, because of the stigma around AIDS, I couldn't acknowledge him, or risk outing myself when no one knew I was positive. It was a very strange and wonderful feeling to be able to finally say hello to him in public.

I said, for the first time outside of his office, "Hi, Dr. Wilson."

He rose from his table and shook my hand. I wanted to say to the other doctors at the table, "This is the man who has helped saved my life, who has coached me through many weird emotional phases of trying to endure HIV, who made me believe that it was okay to think I was going to live, who taught me it was okay to laugh when talking about AIDS, who showed me I have treatment options and who was willing to work with what I told him about how treatment made my body feel."

But I was so shocked at being able to address him at all that I said nothing.

"Hi, Regan, great to see you. Are you going to the Bill Clinton plenary?"

"Absolutely," I said.

"Get there early," Dr. Wilson said. "Clinton can fill even a room of five thousand pretty fast."

"Okay, thanks for the advice," I said. "See you there."

As I walked away from Dr. Wilson down a long hallway of the conference center, I noticed a sign that said "PWA Lounge." PWA stood for "people with AIDS," and the lounge was exactly that—a place to rest, get great food and drink, be massaged, take a nap, have a chiropractic session and converse exclusively with people living with the virus.

The sign at the door stated explicitly that you had to be HIV-positive to enter. I couldn't imagine that anyone would disrespect that, so I was surprised when I was stopped at the door.

"Excuse me, but only HIV-positive people are allowed in here," a man said.

He stared at my badge, which read: "Media." Perhaps he thought I was trying to enter to do a story about the lounge.

"I have HIV," I said.

We stared at each other, and then he said quickly, "Oh, I'm sorry. Come in, come in."

I felt lots of eyes on me as I wandered through a space that looked like a spa and a nightclub combined. People lay sprawled out on low beds in a softly lit area. Others congregated on small clusters of modern furniture, talking and laughing. As I walked by, there was a lull in the conversation. I was a newcomer to the international HIV-positive community, whose members were used to seeing each other yearly at the convention, and my face was unfamiliar.

When I looked around the room, I didn't see disease; I didn't see people with AIDS; I saw beautiful and strong men and women who were very much alive and well.

Over lunch, I sat with some women from Malawi, and some from India, who shared how they'd come together to support each other when their husbands, who had given them the disease in the first place, threw them out of their houses. Left to fend for themselves in countries where it was nearly impossible for women to do that, even with the new micro-lending programs intended to help them become self-sufficient without having to resort to the world's oldest trade, they were fascinated to hear how I was supporting myself and paying for my medicines with no husband. I told them about my job at *POZ* and how lucky I was to be able to afford health insurance, which covered the costs of my treatment. But I also explained that I lived in fear of a day when, because of HIV, I'd get too sick to be able to work, and therefore wouldn't be able to afford health insurance and care. I said that while I was okay for the moment, the balance between my health and my ability to work to make enough money to pay for my life-saving treatment was a fragile one.

"It's easier now, though," I said. "Because I can tell my co-workers when I need to go to the doctor, and because rather than worry silently all the time about AIDS, I get to worry out loud."

They laughed and said that worrying together was much better for us all than worrying alone. Indeed.

While I loved the sanctuary provided by the PWA lounge, it also struck me that there was something very wrong about the idea of it. It seemed weird to be self-quarantined and it was awkward, because if you were hanging out with some people and wanted to put your feet up and slam back a smoothie together, they couldn't join you—unless they too were positive. Anything that makes the HIV community seem "other" is dangerous—because it isolates the community while preventing others from connecting to the very real and present danger of HIV in their own lives.

The hidden nature of the HIV community allows people to maintain their illusion that we aren't normal, thereby perpetuating the idea that only weirdos get AIDS. "It can't happen to me" turns into "I can't believe this happened to me" for tens of thousands a people a year in America and millions of people around the world who remain anonymous. Partly this is because people with HIV don't feel that they can be open about having the disease, which means the world at large rarely sees the HIV community. Therefore, people fear and misperceive what they do not know, and live in denial that people with HIV are just like them. The invisibility of the HIV community means we fail as an incredible tool of prevention: there's nothing like seeing someone who could be you living with HIV to make you realize just that—it could be you.

Until they heard my story, many of my single friends were still sleeping around without condoms because they erroneously believed themselves immune. Incredibly, even after she heard my story, one friend admitted that she wasn't using condoms. When I pushed her to tell me why my story hadn't made her realize that she was at risk, she admitted something that lies, I believe, at our inability to prevent the spread of HIV. Rather than believe me and be forced to change the way she approaches and has sex, she chose to make up a story to establish me as "other" so she could continue to have sex her way. She said that I'd lied about getting HIV from my boyfriend, that I must have done something "extraordinary" to get the virus.

"Like what?" I asked, incredulous.

"Like maybe you were a sex worker or an IV drug user and you just don't want to tell people," she said.

"Or maybe," I suggested, furious, "you just want to believe that because you're too scared or unempowered to protect your own life."

Too many people similarly put themselves in harm's way, vainly thinking that they are "different" from the people who get HIV. But as I looked around the PWA lounge, it was perfectly obvious to me that the virus doesn't know, or care, whether you're black or white or Latino, gay, bi or straight, young or old, male or female or transsexual, rich or poor. As an equal opportunity offender, it comes most easily to those who are most sure of their alleged immunity.

The opening ceremony of the International AIDS Conference was a lot like a rock concert—tens of thousands of people, a giant sound system, multiple JumboTrons. Except Bill and Melinda Gates were onstage instead of leather-clad rockers. About halfway through, I was wandering out to get some fresh air when a tall, handsome man with a shaved head stopped and introduced himself. He told me his name was Carl and that he was HIV-positive. Something about him intrigued me; when he asked if I'd like to have lunch with him the next day at the PWA lounge, I agreed.

When I arrived, he was sitting alone at a table. We talked and shared our histories. When he was younger, he told me, he was attracted to men, but his upbringing prevented him from openly exploring his feelings. So he fought those urges until he couldn't resist anymore. He started doing drugs and ended up dancing in a go-go bar called Bananas. Somewhere in the midst of all of it, he contracted HIV. But eventually, according to him, he rediscovered Jesus—and stopped the men, the drugs and the go-go dancing.

He labeled himself an ex-gay evangelical Christian. He'd started an AIDS ministry at his church, and he was encouraging it to reconsider its stance on AIDS. When not spreading the good word, he delivered pizza.

I told him my story and he listened intently, laying his hand on my forearm as I got choked up when relaying how, after ten years, it felt so good to be talking openly about HIV.

We met several more times, lunching and snacking together. One afternoon, we got side-by-side massages in the lounge and sprawled for hours on the leather couches talking about our lives—forgetting we were two people with HIV, becoming just a man and a woman who liked talking to each other.

Every night of the conference, there were cocktail parties, secret get-togethers of AIDS activists, pow-wow sessions in people's rooms. The media center, where we were all based, was full of thousands of journalists from all over the world—and open all night. I took Carl to one of the sponsor's parties one night; MTV had conducted a HIV documentary video contest for HIV-positive youth. After the short films were shown, the lights went down, the music went up and we danced for hours.

Finally, sweaty and tired, Carl asked if I was ready to go. We ran downstairs while the music throbbed, racing each other to the front door, laughing.

Carl and I found ourselves sitting on a stone wall waiting for a cab. While the wind cooled our hot skin, he reached down and took my hand in his, rubbing it lightly with his other hand. He looked at me.

"I had so much fun tonight. I'm really glad we met," he said.

"Me too," I said.

Although normally a situation like this would have built considerable tension, the air between us was not singing. So I was a little surprised when he leaned in to kiss me. I wanted to believe that he wanted to be with women, but I didn't. I felt as if I was part of a social experiment. My rational mind thought I was helping him to explore heterosexuality, but my subconscious mind knew better: really, I was helping him to face what he was trying so hard to deny—he was gay, even if he thought Jesus didn't want him to be.

We had genuine affection and attraction for each other. We laughed and drank and danced well together. It wasn't that we didn't want to go there. If he had been straight, we might have. But after a kiss totally devoid of any electricity, we said goodnight at the curb and I rode home in the taxi. Because of HIV, I reflected, I was perhaps able to understand in a way I never could have before what it was like to be gay, or black, or an ex-con or anything else that makes you have to struggle to maintain self-esteem while society at large looks down its nose at you.

As someone raised in the Roman Catholic Church who dutifully attended Sunday mass for at least the first seventeen years of my life, I understood Carl's predicament. He didn't want to be kicked out of a group where he felt comfortable. He was being forced by that group to choose between his faith and his desires. To feel a part of something bigger than himself, he chose to subjugate his instincts to follow the rules of organized religion. But it was so sad to me that a place of worship, supposedly offering unconditional love and support to its members, couldn't accept same sex coupling. This, and the way the Church drops you like a hot potato when you get divorced, are two reasons I no longer go to Catholic mass. Because just when you need it the most, the Church kicks you out. Such an approach doesn't seem very Christian or benevolent to me.

Nowhere in the Bible does it say that some things are beyond reproach, forgiveness or tolerance. In the Bible, Jesus befriended lepers, so why couldn't the church embrace people with AIDS— the modern-day equivalent of lepers? And I really couldn't understand how the Church failed to see that as a direct result of faith-based organizations' stance on sex, sex ed and AIDS, the disease continues to spread, even among the most devoted— including members of the clergy itself.

I find it amazing that so many faith-based groups have not found a way to embrace people living with HIV, and that legions of its members, including the pope, refuse to engage in conversations about condoms—a thin piece of latex that allows people to have sex safely. Condoms do not make people have sex; condoms allow people to have the sex they are going to have no matter what, without risking their lives or the lives of others. I just do not understand what the problem is. I understand that the Church links condom use to the promotion of premarital sex, which it does not condone, but given that marriage has become one of the biggest risk factors for contracting HIV (because of the international infidelity rate and married couples' typical reluctance to use condoms, which can imply a breach of monogamy) it seems to me that the Church should rethink its stance.

Abstinence, which was the main focus of sex education under the last Bush Administration, does work, as long as you can keep people from having sex. This proves to be problematic, which is why sex-education curricula promoting abstinence until marriage have been scientifically proven to increase the rate of STD transmission and unwanted pregnancy. Telling kids about sex and its consequences, even arming them with condoms, does not make them get into bed with more partners sooner. In fact, comprehensive sex education delays the onset of sexual activity, which was, last time I checked, about twelve years old.

I am not against abstinence. It's the surest way to keep people from spreading sexually transmitted diseases and from having unwanted pregnancies. I'm a romantic and I love the mutual respect and emotional and physical safety afforded by faithful, loving coupling. But no one has ever been able to keep people from having premarital and extramarital sex. Not our presidents. Not even the popes. Countries such as Australia and Brazil successfully stemmed their AIDS epidemics because they didn't waste time and money trying to keep people from having sex and doing IV drugs; instead, they allowed people to talk about these things without snickering or feeling uncomfortable or flat out lying. In doing so, they empowered people to have sex (and use IV drugs) safely. Only the acknowledgement that people have sex and do drugs, including IV drugs, and the expenditure of time and money to teach people how to do those things safely instead of trying to make them abstain, will stop the spread of AIDS.

When I got home to New Jersey, and sat in a local diner trying to chew a burger and digest the massive emotional, scientific, cultural, political and intellectual overload that was the International AIDS Conference, I couldn't help wondering what the hell I'd gotten myself into. The 26,000 people who attended the conference are not even the tip of an iceberg. Worldwide, 33 million-plus people are HIV-positive. Countless others are trying to save their lives. The problem of AIDS is enormous, and a single person's impact may be inconsequential, no matter how profoundly well intentioned it is or how well it is made.

Thinking of how my life had changed so much in just several months, and exhausted from the conference, I started to cry. Right there in public. But as the salty rivulets burned the tired skin under my eyes, I thought about all the people living with HIV who don't have the time for the luxury of a cry because they're too busy trying to survive. An Argentine friend once told me an expression: *Calaveras no chillan.* Skulls don't cry. I interpreted it to mean that one day, I will be dead and nothing will matter—my empty skull will be unable to shed tears of sorrow, or joy—so I shouldn't waste my life being beaten down and sad; instead, I should enjoy and appreciate all of whatever life I had.

I sighed out some of my fatigue and told myself I'd have plenty of time to sleep when I was dead.

CHAPTER
eighteen

A few months after the International AIDS Conference, one of my mom's good friends, Selden, asked if I would speak about HIV at the Nassau Club, a private club in Princeton. Princeton is hard-core preppy—a land of velvet headbands, Nantucket red pants speckled with tiny lobsters, loafers with no socks and corduroy blazers with leather patches at the elbows. It's not a place you'd ever expect to find or talk about AIDS.

The idea was for me to speak to the members of my community, particularly the old guard, explaining my decision to come forward and educate them about HIV. I imagined that many there would have heard by now about The Situation, and gossiped about it in hushed voices, but I'd been so busy with my new job that I hadn't seen many people I knew socially since my public disclosure.

I'd told the whole world I was HIV-positive, and yet the idea of standing in front of people I grew up with was terrifying. I was equally thrilled and petrified, when my mom called to tell me that by giving people an occasion to hear my story straight from the horse's mouth, and letting them ask questions, I might heighten their comfort with the subject and, ideally, help them rethink their position on AIDS—if it wasn't a benevolent position to begin with.

The morning of the talk, I stood around making polite but nervous conversation with some dear friends who had come.

A woman who walked her dog with my mom touched my shoulder and whispered conspiratorially, "We're so proud of you. You are so brave."

"Thank you," I said, and choked on the words. There was nothing like someone telling you you're brave to jump-start your deepest fears.

I prayed that whatever my HIV status would do to unfavorably color people's perceptions of my character, I would be able to counteract any ill will with my willingness to publicly own up to my mistake and try to inspire other people to make choices that might save their lives.

I went downstairs to the ladies' room to mentally prepare myself. The stalls had white wood lattice doors, just like those in the ladies' room in our country club, where I used to swim and play tennis as a young girl. There were fresh flowers by the sink, and the walls were papered in antique wallpaper. In that tiny respite of civility, I tried to slow my breathing and tell myself that at least this crowd was so well mannered there would likely be no outward signs of their shock and horror.

I called my sister. As always, Tracy gave me a pep talk to enable me to do the seemingly impossible.

When we were younger, we'd watched a war movie together called *Gallipoli*, in which two friends are runners in the trenches in WWI. They'd grown up together, and trained together as competitive runners at university. At the end of the movie, the life of one depends on the speed of the other, who recalls how his coach used to prep him before a race.

His coach would ask him, "What are your legs?"

And the runner would reply, "Steel springs."

"What are they gonna do?" the coach asked.

"Hurl me down the track."

"How fast can you run?"

"Fast as a leopard."

"Well, let's see ya do it, then!"

My sister and I had repeated this conversation to each other umpteen times—whenever the other was afraid to face something we had to do—such as compete in our state field hockey championships, or in Tracy's case, take the bar exam after law school.

"Tracy, I am so scared. I don't think I can go upstairs," I said, while cold water from the faucet ran over the wrist of my hand not holding the phone. I was trying to lower my body temperature, to numb myself into calmness.

"What are your legs?" she said.

"Steel springs," I said, weakly.

"What are they gonna do?"

"Hurl me down the track?" I asked.

"How fast can you run?" she growled firmly.

"Fast as a leopard," I said, closing my eyes and trying to picture surviving the talk.

"Well, let's see ya do it, then!!!" she commanded. And then, "I love you. You'll be fine. Call me when it's over."

I looked at myself in the mirror. Though I felt terrified, I looked surprisingly calm and confident. Perhaps it was resignation. I dried my hands, pinched some color into my wan cheeks and marched up the stairs on the steel springs of my legs.

Upstairs, my mom and I stood around drinking tea awkwardly, wondering how many people would come. More people started to flow through the door, and it seemed as if everyone

I'd grown up with and their parents and their parents' friends would be there. As the who's who of Princeton ate pastries off tiny bone-china plates at linen-clothed tables around the room, I considered making a bolt for the door.

Eventually, the guests took their seats. My mother sat in the back of the room, directly in front of me so I could see her through the sea of curious faces staring at me. Some smiled encouragingly. Perhaps out of pity. Rev. Carl Reimers, who had married Charlie and me spoke about the need for a renewed commitment to AIDS awareness, prevention, testing and treatment. Then I was given an introduction by Selden, who had orchestrated the event. I nearly burst into tears at her kind words. Instead, I took a big swig of ice water and accidentally inhaled a big mouthful of ice. There were several tense moments while I crunched the cubes loudly, trying to clear my mouth so I could speak. The women in the front row stared at me intently from beneath their Palm Beach helmets, doubly secured with hair spray and bobby pins. Their legs were crossed; their clasped hands rested primly on their stockinged knees. I told myself they wanted me to be okay.

Somehow, I managed to get through all the details of how I'd acquired HIV, lived with it in silence for ten years, decided to finally come clean, and do the work I was doing now. I talked for forty-five minutes. Everyone in the room sat stone faced and silent. Were it not for my mother's encouraging nods, I think I would have run screaming from the stares of the people whose expressions I could not read.

When I finished, there was a long pause. And then one of Princeton's most intimidating women started clapping enthusiastically. More joined and soon the room gave me a standing ovation. I almost burst into tears again, but thankfully, Selden, seeing me falter, invited questions. Many hands jabbed the air.

Selden pointed to a tall, elegant woman with a fluff of white hair.

She stood confidently, folding her hands in front of her as she did, and said, "I just want to say that I asked my doctor to give me an AIDS test shortly after I was widowed, and he declined, saying it was unnecessary. I insisted. I told him I was ready to go forward in my life and wanted to be sure I was safe. It made me mad that he seemed shocked that a woman of my age, which is seventy, by the way, was planning on 'getting it on.' I told him to test me and that was that."

The crowd erupted in raucous clapping.

Afterward, people gathered around, hugging me and gripping my arms and hands and kissing my face. My veins felt filled with air rather than tainted blood.

Ironically, now that people are living so much longer and may have good health well into their late seventies, and with the introduction of Viagra and Cialis, many more older people are staying sexually active. As many of them were virgins when they got married, they aren't well versed in the dangers of unprotected sex, nor do they have the experience they need to advocate for the safety of their bodies in the heat of the moment. And because there are so many fewer eligible bachelors relative to the number of older women, there is a lot more overlap between partners.

Which explains why people over the age of fifty are one of the fastest-growing segments of new HIV infection. A complicating factor is doctors' unwillingness to test older people, in part because in small towns like the one in which I grew up, the doctors are members of their patients' social circles and may not feel comfortable diagnosing their friends with HIV. And, many doctors are in the same position as the rest of society—in denial

that certain types of people can get HIV. What puts you at risk
is the thinking that no matter who or what you are, you are immune to HIV.

In the months that followed my talk at the Nassau Club, I got
a bunch of calls and emails from young women whose mothers
had heard me. Some thanked me; others jokingly cursed me for
making their mothers aware of AIDS and ready to talk to them
about safe sex.

My own mother and I learned to speak about sex without
shame, discomfort or embarrassment thanks to HIV. We'd come
a long way, too. It was almost funny to think back on the day
in the '80s, long before I was diagnosed, when she saw a report
about AIDS in the news, called Tracy and me at college and said
we must "never have sex again."

If you had told me then I'd one day be able to talk to my
mom about sex so openly, I wouldn't have believed you. One day,
not long after I started at *POZ*, my mom and I were talking on
the phone on my commute into the city as we did nearly every
day. She said to me, "I don't understand why people get so upset
about condoms. They're like Band-Aids. Or gardening gloves.
They're just a protective device."

And I wished she could have seen my face as it split wide
open in a grin at her analogy.

Last summer, when having lunch with my friend Kathy at her
country club, the conversation turned to AIDS and sex. In between bites of her Waldorf salad, she whispered, "So, what do
you have to do to protect a man's thingy from your infected
hoo-hoo?"

"Hoo-hoo?" I asked.

"Yes, you know, your hoo-hoo," she whispered again, pointing at her crotch with her fork.

"You know, Kathy, it's called a vagina—not a hoo-hoo."

"Oh, I know," she said and flushed, looking around to see if anyone was listening. "It's just that, well, 'vagina' is such an ugly word."

"Have you seen *The Vagina Monologues?*" I asked. My sister and I had, years ago. I remembered how squeamish I'd felt then sitting next to my little sister as the women on stage said "vagina" eighty million times. But as with anything that makes us uncomfortable, if we do it enough, it gets much easier. I decided to share my secret.

"Kathy, I have some homework for you. I want you to say 'vagina' and 'penis' hundreds of times in the next couple of days. You can do it when you're alone in the shower, or the car. You don't have to say it in front of anyone. But you have to say it out loud. Do it and call me in a couple of days and tell me if it's any easier."

She agreed.

She called me a few days later, effusive, as I bagged food in the checkout line at the grocery store. "You are so right!" she said. "I can say it! Penis, penis, PENIS! Va . . . GINA!"

I put my finger over the hole in my phone where the sound came out, as I was in the checkout line of the grocery store and the teenaged boy who was scanning my groceries looked at me wide-eyed.

"Oh, and by the way," I said, looking the teenaged boy right in the eye. "You use a condom to protect a penis from the vagina. And vice versa. You can say 'condom,' can't you?"

HIV has helped me not to be embarrassed when talking about nuanced techniques of oral sex or how to put a condom on safely when you're tipsy, in the dark, without sticking your fingernail through it or pinching your boyfriend's or husband's penis. And I'm not afraid to talk about all those "in between" moments of sex, those moments between kissing each other's mouth off and sliding lips and fingers everywhere before actually having intercourse. Because sex is not just kissing—or intercourse. It's also everything in between. And it is in those in-between moments, when part of your sanity is still intact, when arousal and displaced blood flow have not rendered you hopelessly irrational, that you make the decisions that save, or threaten, your life and that of your partner. That's the stuff we really need to talk about.

After the Nassau Club, I was asked to speak about AIDS at a local prep school. AIDS was attacking people at the other end of the age spectrum, too.

Cheryl, my ex-publisher, had a daughter, Dana, at the local prep school, and together, they had orchestrated my speech, which coincided with "A Day Without Art"—an annual day dedicated to AIDS awareness. It is held in honor of all those lost to AIDS. On this day, museums covered all their art with black shrouds.

Touched that Cheryl and Dana had thought to invite me, I didn't even think about what it meant to speak to a group of children about HIV.

When I accepted the invitation, the administrators at the school asked that I refrain from "talking too much about sex, or condoms." I told them there was no point in my coming to speak to the kids about HIV if I couldn't tell them how not to get the disease. The head administrator said she'd talk with the board and let me know.

She called back and said that I could use the word "condom"

and field some questions about sex if they came up. If it came up? I was talking to five hundred kids between the ages of eleven and eighteen about an STD; the subject of sex was going to come up.

When I arrived on campus, word had gotten around that the "girl with AIDS" was coming to talk that day. The high school boys and girls filing into the pews of the school chapel stared at me as I chatted with teachers and the chaplain.

I gave them the usual story, making a point of saying that I'd gotten the disease through unprotected sex. I didn't care whether or not they thought I was a slut; I cared about keeping them from becoming a statistic: 50 percent of all new HIV infections in the United States are among people under the age of twenty-five.

When I finished, I asked if there were any questions. A young boy who was not yet five feet tall stood up in the balcony, raising his hand in the air.

"Yes?" I said.

"Um, yeah, well, can you tell me, if my girlfriend is going down on me, and some stuff comes out and I have HIV, can she get it by getting it in her mouth?" He shoved his hands down in his pockets and clenched his skinny arms along the length of his slight body. While he waited for my response, his eyes darted around the room anxiously.

I'd been instructed to defer to the chaplain before answering a question.

I turned to him, and raised my eyebrows.

He squinted, tipped his chin to the floor, nodded and made a sweeping motion toward me with both hands; I took it as a sign that it was okay for me to answer the boy.

I had to wait for the snickering to stop before I answered.

"First, I want to thank you for being so brave and asking such a specific question," I said. "This is how you learn to save your life and the lives of other people."

The snickering stopped.

"Secondly, if you are HIV-positive, there is some risk that if your girlfriend performs unprotected oral sex on you, she could contract the virus, though the risk is considered very low, and certainly lower than if you had unprotected anal or vaginal sex."

He was staring intently at me and nodding.

As I answered him, this tiny boy, I tried to imagine him having sex, and could not. I couldn't blame his parents or teachers for thinking that he didn't need to be educated yet about sex. But there he was, telling us that it was happening. He was hungry for answers, willing to be responsible. And he deserved to know the truth.

He hung on my every word.

"Thank you," he said when I finished. And to the great surprise of both of us, the whole school clapped when he sat down.

We give kids way too little credit for being able to handle information about sex. Denial is killing them, and our refusal to share life-saving information with the future generations of the world is as unforgivable as using all their natural resources and creating a global economy that no one can manage.

When I was in seventh grade, I had a crush on a boy, Timmy, who was in my class. One day, he invited me to get off at his bus stop. Timmy said he'd walk me home (he lived two farms away). We jumped off the big yellow bus and sat down on the sunny grass beside the cow fields that led to his house. We sat talking and laughing until we heard a deep, painful moan. He had just reached out for my hand; what might have been intended as a tender squeeze turned into a death grip on my skinny fingers as we saw, at the same moment, two tiny placenta-covered hooves protrude from the vulva of a cow. She was lying on her side, panting and mooing and heaving and writhing while her calf tried to wriggle its way into the world.

We sat in stunned silence as we watched the baby cow tear her open and slip out into the world in a rush of blood and fluid and afterbirth. Exhausted, she flopped her head down on the ground while the calf struggled to break free of the placenta that covered it like an alien pod, desperate for its first breaths of air. Instinctively, the cow picked up her head. It swung like an anvil on her thin, tired neck as she strained her square mouth back toward her baby and ripped the sac open with her teeth so oxygen could fill its lungs. The calf opened up its mouth and gasped at the air.

We did the same.

Suddenly, we noticed we were holding hands.

We jumped apart and leapt to our feet.

"Well, I guess I better walk you home," he said.

"I'm okay by myself," I said.

And he sighed with relief and ran up the road toward his house.

Unbeknownst to us, we'd just gotten a dose of the best birth control and protection against exposure to STDs there is: reality.

CHAPTER
nineteen

In the fall of 2006, I found myself on a plane headed to New Orleans for the "Staying Alive" AIDS conference. This was my first chance to travel not just as a person living with HIV, but as one of a large group of AIDS leaders, advocates, and activists.

It had been many years since I'd last been to New Orleans. The last time, I went with Lyerly and Chase, when we were seniors at Trinity, and stayed at Lyerly's aunt's house for spring break. We'd drunk too much, slept too little, eaten too many oysters at Cooter's Oyster bar and danced our nights into days at Tipitina's (a place that I thought, for years, was called "Tippy Tina's") Years ago, propelled by the invincible feelings of youth, I'd tempted fate. Now I'd come to reckon with it.

As my plane descended to New Orleans, the man seated next to me asked why I was coming to town. He had closely cropped business hair and wore a very expensive bespoke suit.

"I'm the editor of POZ, a magazine for people living with HIV," I said without hesitation. "I'm speaking at an AIDS conference. The conference will look at how we can improve access to care and treatment for those of us with HIV."

Without a blink he said, "That sounds way more interesting than what I'm doing here. I'm in sports marketing and am hoping to convince a potential client to sign with us."

I've learned that the voice with which I deliver the news that I'm living with HIV has a lot to do with how people hear me. If my voice trembles, so does their confidence. If I am unapologetic and strong, they often seem nonplussed.

Later, he passed me in the baggage area, waved congenially and wished me good luck. As I rode to my hotel in the cab, I marveled at how easy something that had previously been so terrifying had become.

The next morning, I turned on the TV and woke up to the sound of Jack LaLanne's voice. The '70s fitness king, bare-chested—and surprisingly well muscled—was standing waist deep in a swimming pool, still pumping iron at the age of ninety-two.

"To die?" he said in between grunts, "that's simple. To live—that's the hard thing."

I agreed entirely with old Jack. I managed to pull myself out of bed and into the shower before setting out to walk along the streets of New Orleans. Taking an early morning walk before I had to speak publicly soothed my nerves and helped me focus. It was also often the only time I had to see many of the cities I visited for work.

It had been almost exactly a year since Hurricane Katrina had unforgivingly pounded New Orleans into a pulp. The part of New Orleans that is its financial lifeblood—the French Quarter/Bourbon Street area—seemed untouched by the deluge (most of it was spared by Katrina's poststorm surge of floodwaters). The streets were still lined with massive palm trees dressed in white lights for the holiday season. Even at nine AM, zydeco music blared from open storefronts and competed with jazz, blues and rock that blasted from clubs, their windows flung wide open despite the unseasonably cool weather. Five and dime stores hawked beads (for those too shy to show some skin and earn them the old-fashioned way), hot sauce and feather boas. I bought handfuls of beads, a mini six-pack of Tabasco and a sapphire blue boa.

Surprisingly, a sense of cheerful resilience permeated the city once better known for its disproportionately high murder rate than for its ability to breed survivors. While it would be unfair, and maybe inappropriate, to compare the spirit of New Orleans in the aftermath of natural disaster to the spirit of New York after the terrorist attack, I couldn't help feeling that there was a similarity in the upbeat defiance of those who had stayed—and those who had returned to the city—after the tragedy of the storm.

Everyone made a point of saying "Welcome to New Orleans" so emphatically that it was surely more than a false-friendly greeting given to those who had come to drink in the debauchery of the town. The people of New Orleans were grateful to have tourists. It seemed the perfect place to assemble four hundred–plus people—many of whom had themselves survived HIV—to talk about how we could go on as a community in the aftermath and bring AIDS' deadly warpath to a halt.

I was scheduled to speak that day at the opening plenary session of "Staying Alive." I'd labored over my remarks the night before and been a nervous wreck all morning.

As others took the stage before me, I surveyed the room. It was full of mostly African Americans. It was also, ironically, the anniversary of the day Martin Luther King Jr. received the Nobel Peace Prize. Listening to others discuss the rights of people with

AIDS to access the life-saving health care they need, I was reminded of the tenets of Dr. King's work and marveled over how similar the gay rights, civil rights and AIDS rights movements were to one another: disempowered communities decided they'd had enough and stood up for their rights to be treated the same as everyone else. And they tried to change the world's perception that they were somehow different, and therefore less deserving.

As I waited for my turn to go on stage, I remembered a Neville Brothers song called "Sister Rosa" about civil rights hero Rosa Parks. The Nevilles dedicated the song to her for being a symbol of "our dignity," what the black community wanted back then and what those of us living with HIV wanted now. It amazed me to see the parallels between how the black community was once treated and how we currently treat people living with HIV. All people want their basic dignity to be respected. It doesn't seem too much to ask, in my opinion.

AIDS is the number one killer of African American women between the ages of 25 and 34. Though African Americans comprise only 13 percent of the U.S. population, they are 48 percent of all new AIDS cases. AIDS is no longer the sole domain of gay white men. Looking out into the audience, it became clear to me that our mutual struggle for survival trumps the difference in our skin color, country of origin, sexual orientation, religion, politics or worldview. Bound together by our bad biology, we break down barriers put up by people who haven't realized the human race is one.

After the meeting, a collection of AIDS activists (who had gathered to talk about how we could bolster our efforts to advocate on behalf of the HIV community on Capitol Hill) were taken on an excursion through Hurricane Katrina's wreckage, still there almost twelve months after she slammed into the Gulf.

As the tour bus trundled into the first affected neighborhood and we got our first glimpse of houses struck by the floodwaters, there were gasps of disbelief. The bus was filled with agitated chatter as we looked at another example of what can happen when the government responds too slowly, incorrectly or not at all to an obvious, massive, and crippling force of nature.

The big bus swung past houses with watermarks above the tops of their first-story windows. Giant trees lay toppled on crushed roofs, exposing the insides of the houses to the elements—ironically, a benefit, as mold spread less in houses with exposure to sunlight and air. Cars sat crazily on top of other houses as if even they had tried to escape the storm surge—and everywhere, there were Dumpsters and front-end loaders poised for cleanup, but in many of the neighborhoods, not a soul was to be found. Looking at street after street after street of devastation it was hard to figure out even where to begin to start picking up the pieces. Add to that the fact that there was no power, it was no wonder it looked like the floodwaters had receded just a week ago.

In the wealthy white neighborhoods, order had been restored. But the poorer parts of town were still an abject mess.

Adding to the eerie Pompeii-ish feeling was the legion of dead oak trees throughout the affected areas. Of four thousand trees planted in one park, one thousand of them were killed by the floodwaters—the salt was fatal. Their dead, leafless branches pointed up to the sky like the machine-guns carried by the National Guard soldiers who were posted to keep order in abandoned areas. The guards weren't too busy; no one went into the empty parts of town after dark.

Hundreds of migrant workers had come to live in tent villages while rebuilding the city, and there were federally funded, ad hoc trailer parks built behind chain-link fencing—temporary housing for displaced residents. There was no point in many of the residents of New Orleans coming back, as they had no place to stay while they rebuilt, and no money to literally clear the slate even if they could manage to get their hands on the funds to rebuild their lives.

The loud banter that had filled the bus at the start of the tour died down as we got deeper into the area of destruction, so massive that it was hard to fathom. Nearly a third of the city was gone or uninhabitable. And as we got closer to ground zero—the Ninth Ward, where the waters first burst through the levee, it got harder and harder to look out the window.

Just as I was thinking *This can't possibly be America*, I saw a building spray-painted with big black letters. They read: BAGHDAD.

All the houses bore a colorfully painted X—a sign from relief workers to indicate which unit had checked the house, the date, the number of survivors and the number of dead. Some were marked "NE," which meant "not entered." Precarious buildings on the verge of collapse had been avoided.

On one house, there was a note spray-painted in two-foot letters: "Blk K-9 under porch." Indicating that there was a black dog trapped underneath the steps. Dead animals were not reflected in the body counts.

On the outside of other homes, people had written other notes to loved ones: "Billy, gone to Tennessee. Call me. I love you."

On still others, there were pleas for help: "Need money to rebuild. Please call with donations." And always, a phone number—ten digits—the only thing left of a whole life washed away.

The bus stopped and we got out. The only signs of life were beautiful white egrets tip-toeing through the debris. I looked in the doorway of a house and tried to imagine that it was my own. I tried to imagine whether I would want to roll up my sleeves and start cleaning off the river's mud, which coated everything like plaster, or if I'd want to leave it all behind like a bad dream.

More than anything, I felt scared and ashamed to live in a country whose government could let its citizens down like this. After the storm, the federal government had done little to rebuild the city; nearly a year later, few of the residents who'd lost their homes had been able to return. I had become somewhat familiar with the terror and anger engendered by knowing that your country had decided your life wasn't worth saving. Before I was diagnosed with HIV, I never really worried about health insurance, disability acts, the price of meds or privacy laws. But after becoming HIV-positive and imagining my privacy being breached over this subject, or being denied health or life insurance, I knew all too well the impact the government had on my quality of life.

I had seen what the government did, and didn't do, to people with HIV in the beginning of the epidemic and I was now at their mercy, like everyone else with AIDS. When the federal government knows there are life-savings AIDS medicines, and can afford to pay for and dispense them, yet people are dying while on waiting lists for the federal AIDS Drug Assistance Program or in prisons and jails because the government won't allow them access to their treatment, it's hard not to question their approach—and motives. There are a million excuses used for why we can't get prisoners who are living with HIV their medicines, but if you ask me, they should be one of the easiest groups to administer information and care to—given that they live in a federal- or state-funded institution all under one roof.

At *POZ*, I got letters from inmates almost daily. I heard firsthand how even in prisons or jails where people had access to medicines to treat HIV, they struggled to take their medicines as prescribed; without food and water, the drugs can be very hard on your stomach. Many prisoners told me that they couldn't tolerate the medicines because they couldn't get food to take with them.

As we boarded the bus to head back to the conference site, the air was silent. People had stopped shaking their heads. We were just numb and confused. How could this happen in America? In my neighborhood, a house goes up in a matter of months. I'd heard that the people displaced from the poorest areas wondered out loud about whether it had been the city's—or the federal government's—intention to wash them all away so that the city could have a fresh start and turn their streets and homes into a pristine park. Standing in the Ninth Ward, it seemed true. How else could you explain the utter standstill and neglect?

It was upsetting to see our country's willingness to fight and help the rest of the world while our own country suffers. Just as it was hard to watch America send money and meds overseas to fight AIDS through the President's Emergency Plan for AIDS Relief (PEPFAR), when I know Americans are dying at home.

In my first years at POZ, George W. Bush was president, and his largesse when it came to fighting AIDS did not extend to his fellow Americans despite a skyrocketing need. In 2006 alone, the estimated number of new HIV cases was later shown to be 40 percent higher than previously stated.

I wouldn't take back a penny of the international support the U.S. government has given, mostly to Africa, for AIDS. Lord knows, I want us to help everyone in need. But it is time for the American government, media and people to wake up to the fact that AIDS is definitely not under control in the United States.

At least 3 percent of D.C. residents have HIV or AIDS. People are dying while on AIDS Drug Assistance Plan waiting lists, and people are still diagnosed with AIDS after repeatedly going to the doctor with symptoms of HIV infection for years. In these circumstances, we can't say that AIDS is under control here at home.

I have to wonder if our foreign adventures are only a diversion to keep us from focusing on the horror in our own backyard. Seeing what had happened to people in Katrina's aftermath, many of whom were HIV-positive, I understood more fully that the enemy in the war on AIDS was not only viral but also ethical, political and socioeconomic.

We drove past a center for children living with HIV/AIDS in New Orleans, abandoned, crumbling and cordoned off, the watermark between the first and second floors. Some of the children had been saved, but their medical records and personal histories had been washed out to sea with the other debris, and what had been known about them was now gone. So were the children themselves—no one knew where they'd ended up.

Remembering the warnings and the resistance of the people of New Orleans to leaving their homes and their belongings made me think about how people are similarly unwilling to hear the truth about the danger of AIDS. We tell people again and again that it is real, and that it can come for them if they don't take the necessary precautions. Yet, as with those people who sat defiantly on their front porches even as the rain began to beat down on their roofs, there seems to be a similar, almost arrogant level of denial about AIDS. How much proof do we need before everyone realizes that anyone who has ever had unprotected sex—even once—is at risk for having contracted HIV and should get tested?

When people ignore nature and are too afraid to look at the truth, when they have false optimism about their ability not to be struck down by the same thing that has taken away 25 million people before them, you almost can't feel sorry when they are hit by the brunt of nature's cruelty. There are some people, like those in New Orleans prior to Katrina's onslaught, who heeded the warnings, understood the danger and would have protected themselves but didn't have the power, or the money. I think about the stories I've heard from HIV-positive women from other nations who said they worried about their husband's fidelity and suspected he was sleeping around, but didn't have the power to insist that he wear a condom because to do so was to accuse him of infidelity—an accusation that could result in a beating, or a divorce. With both AIDS and natural disasters, there are people who can't get out of harm's way because they lack the resources to save themselves.

The next day, still recovering from the demolition I saw, I had lunch by myself in a restaurant. I needed to step away from everything to catch my breath—and I needed to be free of the conference to run *POZ* remotely. I ordered a crab salad and was talking on my phone with my managing editor Jennifer when two women, sisters, having lunch at the table beside me overheard my conversation and asked me what I did.

I told them directly and nonchalantly, newly liberated by my casual approach, and they listened, enthralled. As with the man on the plane, it was liberating no longer to be ashamed to admit casually and publicly that I am living with HIV.

I asked, "Why are you here in New Orleans?"

"Well," said one woman pointing at the other one, "my sister here has a son and he's playing in a big high school football game in the Superdome."

The women and I chatted for a while, then they paid their bill and said good-bye.

As they were walking away, one of the women suddenly stopped, turned, stared at me and with a dramatic swipe of her arm, removed her hat, and then, with a flourish—her hair.

"You know what?" she said to me defiantly, "I have breast cancer and I am a survivor, like you, and if you can say you have HIV I can say I have cancer and I don't have to wear this itchy wig." Her sister and I looked at each other, and at the woman standing there clutching her hair. I stood up and shook her hand. She thanked me with a hearty hug and asked me to wish her son good luck at the football game. I told her I'd look for her beautifully bald head in the crowd.

WINTER 2007–SPRING 2009

CHAPTER
twenty

I returned to New Jersey after the "Staying Alive" conference and things started to settle down. I traveled to Santa Fe to see my family for Christmas. It was amazing to see my parents enjoy being grandparents.

After dinner one night, Tracy asked if I would give her little boy a bath. We filled the tub with hot, soapy water and plunked him into it. As I scrubbed his back gently with a SpongeBob SquarePants—well, sponge—he giggled and blew bubbles and made me promise I wouldn't get soap in his eyes. To go from feeling like a filthy untouchable to being someone who could be trusted to wash a baby with her bare hands brought me back to life in a way that's hard to describe. As we filled toy boats with legions of tiny rubber aliens, and he stared at me with clumpy wet eyelashes, I made a silent promise to myself to do whatever I could to make sure his was a generation not devastated by HIV.

Things leveled off at work, too. I'd broken through my fear of my public speaking, had met a good deal of the power crew in the AIDS community and was slowly earning my place among them. I could now see AIDS through the various lenses—political, scientific, economic and cultural—through which it was perceived and misperceived. I enjoyed focusing again on the magazine and website, and hunkering down with my staff, a group of sharp and passionate people who were determined to change people's minds about AIDS, and who had also become my good friends. It was such a joy to work with people who shared my passion for using journalism to try to reshape people's thinking. Many of them had been doing that for years before I came to POZ; others were fresh recruits, but no less impressive in their passion for putting the power of the pen to good use, and no less determined to serve the community of people living with HIV for whom reading POZ and poz.com were part of their lifestyles.

In the summer of 2007, after six months of relative calm, it was time to get on the road again; the U.S. State Department sent me to the Pacific Rim to speak about AIDS stigma and how we might fight it. They planned a tour through Taiwan, Vietnam and Australia that I'd follow en route to the International AIDS Conference in Sydney.

My first stop was Taiwan. The Taiwanese people love Americans. They give you the peace sign and smile and stare and sometimes follow you for a little while along the crowded streets. I was hosted in Taipei by the American Institute in Taiwan, as we have no embassy there.

Prior to my arrival in Taipei, a memo had been circulated about my coming visit, and soon word spread around the institute that many employees would not come to work the day I was to visit. When I arrived at the institute, I was ushered into the office of my host, Nicholas Papp, Cultural Affairs Officer for the Public Affairs Section of the American Institute. Over tea, he acknowledged that this had happened, but said I should not worry; the institute had brought a doctor in to educate the employees. They had all come to work, having come to understand that I posed no risk to their health.

Even as we sipped tea and he tried to shrug off the grim reality, curious faces poked into the room to get an eyeful of the American with AIDS.

Clearly, stigma, fear and misinformation ran as deeply there as in the United States. I was distraught that education about AIDS was almost nonexistent. Taiwan was a nation of people who wore masks against the cancerous pollution and avian flu, and who were screened by a heat sensor at the airport upon their return to the country, so that anyone carrying SARS could be stopped. How could they be so unaware of the lack of risk posed by casual contact with people living with HIV? Like many countries in the Pacific Rim, Taiwan had a budding AIDS epidemic that no one wanted to talk about, but people had heard it was happening. Which perhaps explained their irrational fear.

My first day in Taiwan, I spoke through a translator to a group of people at the American Institute. They stared stoically as I told my story, and I wondered how much of what I was saying was being relayed accurately. I talked about how critical it was for people living with HIV not to feel physically or socially shunned, and how it meant so much to me when people touched and hugged and kissed me to show they did not fear me.

At the end of my speech, the room stood and applauded and then moved, en masse, to the front of the room to request my business card. One young man asked in English, "May I give you a hug?" I said that of course he could, and as he squeezed me carefully in his arms, he looked over his shoulder, perhaps to drink in the approval of the crowd. I felt a little like a baby alligator in the touch tank at an aquarium. And that he was the brave one who was willing to be first to touch the deadly creature.

Seeing that he survived touching me, others followed suit. I was hugged and squeezed and kissed to the point where I began to feel claustrophobic, but I couldn't bring myself to push them away after convincing them how necessary human touch is to people living with HIV. We took many pictures, with the crowd frantically reconfiguring after each shot like clowns in a VW so everyone could get a turn to sit squished up against the woman with AIDS. I slung my arms around my new friends and smiled encouragingly at the few older people who stood warily at the back of the room, watching others make the transformation from fear to acceptance but not ready to be a part of it.

After my talk, a man named Hank, wearing a tight black shirt and artfully torn blue jeans, and who had a face like a mischievous child, tugged on my arm and with the help of the translator, let me know that he too was living with HIV. He smiled widely while pointing at me, then at himself, then back at me, over and over again. He seemed filled with incredulity that we shared a similar disease, though everything else about us was different. There was something gleeful in his revelation, as if he was so glad to no longer be alone that he forgot the tragedy of what we both faced.

He came to my next talk, and my next. He seemed fascinated to watch me become a tiny bit more comfortable every time I told the same stories, in front of new faces. He was a floral designer, an artist, a man given to great bursts of colorful expression, and it had been killing him not to be able to tell his friends or family. He so desperately wanted to.

At the Taipei Salon—a hip cultural phenomenon in the capital city, sponsoring lectures and discussions on contemporary
issues—an old man stood up slowly and asked how people in developing nations are supposed to choose between paying for food
and HIV treatment. Without either, they will die, but without
food they will die faster he pointed out. "How would you recommend they make that choice?" the old man asked politely but
with a twinge of bitterness.

As I struggled to say something to indicate that even I, the
well-fed American with health insurance, understood this was
an impossible choice, there was an awkward silence followed by
a huge flash of light in the windows and then a head-cracking
crash of thunder.

"I guess that's a question that can only be answered up
there," I said, pointing at the heavens that had grumbled and
cried through most of my trip to the Far East. I wondered if I had
offended people. Many of them were Buddhists, and I wasn't sure
whether Buddha lived in the sky or in a more earthly realm. But
I think they got the point.

Prior to appearing at the Taipei Salon, I had asked Hank if
he wanted to join me on stage and share his story. Quite unex-
pectedly, he took the plunge. At the Salon, he sat beside me and
when it was his turn, stood proudly and spilled his truth. As he
spoke, he seemed to get taller, his chest expanded, and when
he was finished, everyone stood and clapped thunderously. I've
seen Miss Americas cry less dramatically than Hank did at the
response he got for his display of extraordinary bravery.

After we spoke, a few people hung back to talk to Hank and
me. A young, reed-thin woman with dreamy eyes said she was
worried about her friend; he had recently been diagnosed with
HIV but was too afraid to go to the doctor or start taking medications, and she was terrified he was going to die. As she spoke

in a warbling voice, I spied a slight, hip young man standing in the corner and looking defiantly in our direction. I took a chance and asked the wisp of a girl, "Is that him?"

Nervously, she glanced over her shoulder and stared at her friend.

"Yes," she said.

"Well, tell him I will think he's very brave if he comes and talks to me. I will keep his secret, and help him get better."

The Taiwanese boy, who couldn't have been older than seventeen, came over, and standing with his hands thrust into his pockets, stared at me with eyes that seemed to be barely held in their sockets by the tissue-thin layer of skin surrounding them. He spoke no English, so I looked directly at him but spoke to his girlfriend.

"Tell him the medications will make him better and without them he will die," I said. "He doesn't have to fear them. The government will give them to him for free and he doesn't have to tell anyone he's taking them. Tell him he can live to be an old man if he stops fearing the doctor."

She translated in a heated, tinny voice that soared and sunk dramatically. I didn't understand a word she said but it was clear she was imploring him to hear her. He listened without taking his eyes away from mine.

When she finished, I asked what she thought he was thinking. She shrugged. In response, the boy removed his hands from his pockets, raked them through his spiky, ebony hair and let them hang limp by his side. Then he nodded. Slowly but emphatically. She exhaled visibly and smiled at me.

The boy reached out his hand and offered it to me to shake. With his other hand, he pulled his cell phone from his pocket and indicated he wanted to take a picture of the three of us. I grabbed each of them under an arm and they each made the peace sign with one hand. In Taiwan, asking to have your picture taken with someone is a gesture of respect.

On the other side of the stage, Hank had finished talking to a bunch of people who took turns pumping his fist up and down with congratulatory words. I introduced him to my new young friend and they spoke passionately together. I smiled and stepped back, leaving the two HIV-positive Taiwanese men who had been pulled into their truth by the fact that I shared mine.

It was fantastic to think that this was how it could happen. As in the Breck shampoo commercial from the '70s, I'd told two friends, and they'd told two friends, and so on and so on until maybe someday the whole world of people living with HIV will have come forward unabashedly to disclose, and ask for the re-spect and support they deserve.

I left the hall where we'd spoken, opened the door to a wall of chest-squeezing heat and stumbled out onto the curb. A part of me felt like a vampire near daybreak; the act of adding new re-cruits had sapped some of my vital life force, but I was so grateful that the ranks of the disclosed were growing. Like dominos, my fears fell over and in doing so, they toppled over my neighbor's fears, who knocked down their neighbor's fears. And so on and so on and so on.

At my first talk in Taiwan, I met a woman named Nicole who in-vited me to visit the orphanage she ran called Harmony Home—a refuge for children orphaned by parents who died of AIDS. Some of the children were positive and some were not; all had lost their parents to AIDS and had nowhere else to go. But even those not living with the virus weren't welcome into anyone's home; by as-sociation with their parents who died of AIDS, the children were unwanted and reviled. Nicole was a one-woman army who was aided by a small group of kind-hearted students and some older people, some also HIV-positive, who sought shelter at her orphanage in return for helping with the babies. The children slept many to a room and crawled, teetered and ran around two floors of brightly lit, cheerful rooms that were protected with rubber flooring that locked together like puzzle pieces and smelled like the back of a soccer mom's minivan. Everything was sticky.

She told me that the neighbors around the orphanage wanted it to close down. They feared for their lives and the value of their real estate and were lobbying local politicians to evict the residents of Harmony Home.

Fortunately for those in the orphanage, Nicole was as savvy as she was tireless; she'd befriended a high-powered local female politician and was doing a great job getting press about the plight of her orphanage.

She said it would help if we could discuss their work during the many appearances I had scheduled during my one-week stay. And we did. Every chance we had, we used Harmony Home as a local example of how stigma makes it incredibly difficult for people with HIV to survive. Taking away someone's dignity by treating them as if their life is not worth living is bad enough; being so afraid of someone that you take away their housing and medical care is unforgivable. And it happens every day, all over the world, to people living with HIV. I remembered how I feared that my landlord would kick me out of the barn where I live in New Jersey. I knew what the residents of Harmony Home faced. It is terrifying to think that because of HIV you could be homeless. The threat of losing your home or shelter is one the most frightening fates imaginable, and there have been many studies that show a direct link to the security of people's homes and how well they are able to fight the disease. Put people with AIDS on the street and you won't be able to care for them, and isolated from their support systems, they are more likely not to take their treatment out of desperation and depression, and engage in practices that further the spread of HIV. Ironically, the best thing for people who fear those with HIV is to ensure that they are in care and not out on the streets.

Of course, all of this seemed so abstract until I wound up at Harmony Home's staircase, removed my shoes and stepped inside the crayon-colored sanctuary.

Inside, I was greeted by a flock of knee-high kids in summer play clothes who, upon seeing me, dragged me down to the floor and offered me pieces of candy—some half-chewed straight from their own mouths. They climbed into my lap, touching my hair with sugar-coated fingers.

Language is not a barrier for children. They made their desires perfectly clear. We toured their rooms, of which they were very proud, and listened to music, and played with balls and had juice and ice cream. Some of the children had been adopted by Westerners and were waiting for the paperwork to be processed so they could go to America. Others would probably come of age in the orphanage. Some of the women who cared for them had worked as prostitutes, others were students and some were international relief workers.

A small girl in a puff of a pink dress offered me cup after cup of orange juice. We clapped and sang and posed for pictures together. I wanted to take all of them home with me, but I could see that as long as they stayed with Nicole and in their cheerful sanctuary, they might be okay. I promised myself I would return one day and take a child if I could.

The next day, I visited a second orphanage squirreled away on the second floor of an office building in downtown Taipei. No one in the rooms below the orphanage knew that upstairs there were roomfuls of HIV-positive babies, or babies who'd lost their families to AIDS, because the babies didn't make a peep. They barely moved. They were too despondent to cry.

I can't mention the name of the orphanage, or its wonderful director, for fear that it would get kicked out of its secret space. Unlike Nicole, who had been successful at engaging people and the press to help her fight to keep her housing, the woman who ran the smaller orphanage was too overwhelmed by caring for the kids to have the time or energy to lobby for acceptance of her work.

When I arrived, she gave me a thick red rubber apron to wear. "To protect the babies," she said. It seemed unclear how an apron could shield them from anything. They already had HIV, and it made my stomach sweat, but I put it on politely and peered into the first crib. Inside, there was a tiny child with tufts of wild black hair lying on his back, staring at the ceiling.

"What's his name?" I asked.

"Benny," she said.

"Hello, Benny," I whispered into the crib. His head didn't turn to see me.

"Is he okay?" I asked.

"Well, a lot of the children have had so little interaction with people that they don't respond," she said.

I called to him again but I don't think he knew his name.

I picked him up and carried him down to the floor, placing him face up on my bent knees so he could see my face. His eyes roamed around and then he seemed to see me. His mouth moved and twisted and I smoothed his crazy hair down with my hands.

"Hello, Benny," I said.

He wriggled and extended a tiny hand. I held it and jiggled him around. I searched his face for a sign of pleasure, but he seemed only surprised.

The director said she was working on a program that would

enable the babies to spend the weekend with older couples so that they would get some love and attention. It was clear that lying alone on their backs hour after hour with nothing but a white ceiling to stare at was making them catatonic.

We pulled them out of the cribs one by one and let them sit or lie together on the floor. But save for two kids who had been handled regularly, they seemed to have all but given up their life—even before it began.

CHAPTER
twenty-one

A week later, I landed in Hanoi, Vietnam.

The heat in Hanoi is an entity. It waits for you outside the revolving glass door of your intensely refrigerated, all-too-Americanized hotel that does its best to make you feel as if you are comfortably at home. Step out of the hotel door and the Vietnamese summer engulfs you like a clutching maiden aunt; your skin instantly beads with anticipatory moisture, as if your flesh, fearing spontaneous combustion, wets itself in defense against the fiery hot climate—even at night.

Vietnam takes you backward in time.

The country has changed little since the days when the U.S. military rumbled through the rice paddies, spreading liquid fire in the trees, scorching huts made from rushes, as we tried in vain to identify and fight an uncountable, invisible enemy. Strangely, the Vietnamese people seemed welcoming; it was only when I met a pair of eyes set deeply in a wrinkled face that I felt a twinge of animosity. There were not so many older people in Vietnam. When I asked why, I was told, "Because the Americans killed them all." Wandering through the streets of Hanoi, or the small villages that lie along any of the roads leading to the coast, the sights were very much the same as those the American GIs saw when they were here. There were lots of tiny, brown people sitting on overturned buckets, selling sweating fruit in DayGlo colors. There were chickens, old women with bowed sticks over their shoulders carrying stacks of lettuce heads, and water buffalo swishing flies off their haunches with tails like whips.

The only hints of modernity were the long rows of rubber boots along the newly paved road separating the freshly erected Hyundai and Bausch & Lomb factories from chartreuse fields of rice. The shiny legions of latex were a sign of progress; they prevented the leeches that live in the subaquatic crops from affixing themselves to those who have jobs building new cars (or sunglasses or solar panels or bricks) as they walk home through the paddies in which they once labored in the unthinkable heat.

As I walked down the sweltering streets, I tried to picture my dad here, as a young marine. He had come before the war, with marine intelligence. Later, during the war, both of his brothers, Jimmy and Harold, were in Vietnam, too. I wondered if my dad, stomping through the jungles, ever imagined he'd get married, have a daughter, then have her contract HIV and follow him back to Vietnam to fight a different war—against as fierce and as invisible an enemy.

My dad had gone to Annapolis, and, after graduating, had gone into the Marine Corps. I remember finding his "dress blues" in the attic one day as a child. I'd put on his navy blue blazer with buttons polished to a bright gold sheen and inhaled the familiar smell of my father, faint on the coat, so many years after he wore it last. He'd served as an officer for years until blood sugar problems forced him to leave the service. Planning, as he was, to be a career officer, I think the transition to the private sector initially hard for him. But he used the leadership skills and finely tuned sense of duty and ethics he learned in the military and they had, in turn, led him to great success in business. Our relationship grew closer as I aged, and as my jobs got increasingly tougher, I relied more and more on his advice. He'd share bits of wisdom such as: as a leader, you don't have to be well liked but you have to be respected. He said: if people respect you, they'll often like you, too.

I never knew whether his ferocity, unflagging work ethic and raw toughness were part of his core fabric, or whether life had tempered him that way. And I never knew whether I had inherited his toughness, or he had instilled it in me by the way he brought me up. But I knew one thing: he'd made me pretty damn tough. Luckily, I'd also inherited my dad's other side—his sensitive, artisitic, romantic side—that serves, for us both, as a welcome respite from our moments of maintaining a stiff upper lip. Wandering among the Vietnamese people, looking at their sun-wizened faces, I tried to picture having to shoot them, point blank. I couldn't imagine what you had to have inside to do that. Maybe fear of what would happen if you didn't follow your superior's orders. But at the end of the day, it was still you pulling the trigger. For his sake, I was glad my dad had never seen actual combat. But he looked people in the face when he was there, knowing the very real possibility that one day, it might be his job to kill them.

When the Americans were last in Vietnam, in force, we tried to identify those members of society who were trying to kill us. The challenges of the war in Vietnam were many; one of them was that the enemy was uncountable, and often appeared in the form of a woman, or a small child. I reflected that if only people would see the truth, they would realize that AIDS is carried by innocent-looking hosts as well. How many of the people staring at the tall, blond American strolling down the streets believed I had the potential to be as deadly as the other Americans who had come here years ago?

*   *   *

I was staying at the Hanoi Hilton. Except for the almond-eyed
women who brought my fresh laundry every day (folded into im-
possibly tiny origami-esque bundles) and the clusters of lychee
fruit piled beside the bed, it could have been a Hilton anywhere
in the world. If you'd asked me before I'd spent fourteen days in
Asia whether I would have preferred a facsimile of home or a
place that afforded the experience of living locally, I would have
said the latter. But traveling as I was on a mission that thrust me
daily into uncomfortable positions, I was grateful to return each
night to a place that reminded me I would, before too long, be on
my way home to my own bed.

In Hanoi, there is a lot of traffic—cars, bikes, motorbikes,
rickshaws, pedestrians, scooters—and no traffic control. There
are no road signs, no lights, no stop signs, no rules of the road.
Everyone has the right of way, all the time. People perched atop
and hunched inside metal vehicles move in a constant stream in
all directions, meeting at intersections of sometimes as many as
six streets, gently swaying and pausing and accelerating around
one another so that everyone gets where they're going without
ever having to stop. Most people wear masks over their faces to
filter the foul air, and the women, in sleeveless cotton dresses,
wear gloves past their elbows. I was daunted by the fast stream
flowing by, but the women at the hotel had given me the name
of a place to have lunch and I was excited at the possibility of an
hour of quiet by myself with a book and some real Vietnamese
spring rolls.

To cross the road, you have to step off the curb and move
slowly and steadily through the melee. If you run, or stop, you
risk getting run over. There is a lyrical beauty to the movement of
so many people hurtling down the road, inches from each other,

eyes fixed meditatively ahead while their feet and hands jerk and stab at pedals and handlebars and steering wheels, gliding past and through one another like pieces of a river. In the beginning, I just couldn't do it, couldn't trust that everyone would heed my passage. I just couldn't let go and become part of the mass of humanity around me. I couldn't step off the curb.

I was reminded of so many decisive moments that I'd known with Jody—and since saying good-bye to him: to believe or not believe the invigorating idealism of his youth and his sagelike wisdom; to trust, or not, a piercing love; to release, or not, out-dated versions of myself; to dive with him into the river, or to stay in the boat; to take, or decline, the job at *POZ*; to guard my silence around my HIV status or to just let go in the face of fear and the unknown and speak my truth.

As I stood there on the edge of the road, sweating, a young Vietnamese girl noticed me wavering. She took my hand and pulled me with her into the traffic. I closed my eyes, feeling the hot fumes of scooter exhaust on my legs, sensing car antennae sing by millimeters from my face. Her tiny hand was as bony as the chicken feet sold in buckets by the roadside. I held on tight, frightened that she'd slip away, worried that I'd crush her fingers. I stepped deliberately and slowly, reasoning that at least I was tall and blonde and therefore maybe easier to see. When we reached the far side of the street, she vanished into the foot traffic before I could even thank her. And suddenly, as had happened so many times since he drowned, I felt Jody's presence.

Calmed by the feeling of Jody being with me in spirit, I wandered dreamily past storefront after storefront of people sitting on miniature plastic chairs, eating from plastic bowls, some watching a fuzzy TV in the back of the store, some sitting on the filthy sidewalk tinkering with the gears of a bicycle or the engine of a small motorcycle.

And then, suddenly, I saw the sign for the restaurant I was searching for.

After lunch, while starting to make my way home to the hotel, I realized I felt unwell. My body was feeling the effects of being under stress, in sweltering countries, constantly surrounded by strangers, always having to be "on." I'd had trouble eating; my medicines take away my appetite and I couldn't find any of my comfort foods in the land of lychees and chicken boiled in hot oil. So far, the only familiar food I'd found was cornflakes. But I felt fueled by an energy no food could produce. I was driven in part by fear—that there is too little being done to fight the global pandemic, that too many will get sick and die, that I will die before I make any significant difference, that governments and people will never be able to see through the thick cloud of stigma around AIDS to deliver the resources and compassion positive people need. But in part I was driven by sheer joy and awe that I had ended up in a place where I could try to solve these problems firsthand every day. So I ate a bowl of cornflakes back at the hotel and sucked it up.

The next day, having traveled to the coast by minibus with my guide and translators—stopping along the way to eat a chicken that was killed, much to my dismay, on the spot when we ordered it—I awoke in a small hotel in the town of Haiphong that sits near Ha Long Bay.

Looking out my window, I nearly fell into a trance watching a man swim laps methodically in a pool. In the distance, the heavy metal arms of cranes reached for cargo that had been shipped in through the Gulf of Tonkin—a body of water still peppered with live mines put there by the Americans.

I had gone on a boat ride the day before, chugging through strange rock formations with eroded bases that appeared to float magically on top of the water. I'd crawled into grottoes, eaten lunch at a floating fish market, and bought a strand of black pearls. I'd been served breakfast by an exquisite woman in a long white satin gown and a half moon of satin and beads atop her ebony hair. Vietnam was so foreign and fascinating I'd had trouble composing a speech for that morning's appointment with the local Communist government.

So when the van came to collect me, I asked to sit in the back so I could think about what I would say to that morning's audience of positive people, people affected by HIV, people who worked at NGOs, politicians, health officials and government workers.

We pulled into a gated and guarded compound of yellow buildings. Schoolchildren flew across the yard, herded by older women with sharp voices. I was taken to an office that fulfilled my imagination's rendering of where a local Communist Party official might sit. It was windowless, with a big steel desk and a slowly rotating ceiling fan; several filing cabinets and maps; no photos, flowers or anything personal.

Several people emerged, three men and a woman, in drab, serious clothing. They shook my hand and bowed and we were directed to an L-shaped arrangement of low leather couches and given hot tea. I spoke, through my translator, and they answered back formally, politely, briefly. It was clear that it wasn't their idea that I come, but they seemed far happier to receive me than I'd expected and far more open-minded than I thought they would be. Even when I spoke of the importance of their addressing IV drug users and sex workers, and talked about approaches to prevention education and harm reduction tactics that might help these groups, they continued to nod. I could tell that they wanted to help, wanted to try to keep AIDS at bay in their backyard. I felt that they appreciated the American money being sent through PEPFAR and they believed that what I was telling them would help protect their local constituents.

The party leader was soon to be up for election for a more important position, and if I understood the translator properly, he saw helping people living with AIDS as a way to endear him to voters.

After having tea with the officials, I spoke to a group of about one hundred people, while the school children peered through the windows, listening intently to the translation.

Afterward, we drove in silence four hours back to Hanoi, my face pressed against the hot glass of the window as we sped past the thousands of squares of green rice fields peppered with small children on top of water buffaloes or trudging through the ankle-deep water.

Back in Hanoi, I ate dinner at a restaurant called Bobby Chin's frequented by ex-pats. It is owned by the eponymous celebrity chef and sits on the edge of the man-made lake in the center of Hanoi. Climbing down from my rickshaw, I stood for a moment by the still, dark water. And then I turned and walked into the bar glowing with low orange lighting through strand after strand of live white roses suspended from the ceiling. Relieved that I'd survived having breakfast with the Communists, I ordered a celebratory martini and toasted the courage of the local political leaders I'd met that morning, grateful to know that people I'd never have imagined would confront AIDS openly had the ability to do just that.

It was only when I was on another plane, headed to Sydney via Singapore, that I began to get my head around what I'd experienced so far on my journey. I am not an intrepid traveler. I would like to be, like to say I that am; I hope it is something that I might grow in to. But on that maiden trip to the Pacific Rim, I was uncomfortable for much of my time there. My walk was stiff, my back and jaw tense, my smile affixed with a grim determination. I wouldn't be able to truly relax until I was home again.

I once read that to rouse an echo you have to stand away from the wall. If you are too close and speak and wait for sound to bounce back to you, it won't. I think traveling can be like that—when you're right in the thick of a ring of bright-faced Vietnamese girls swirling around you all colors and pigtails and tiny fingers like miniature crab claws gripping your clothes— their mouths and eyes begging you to buy a fan, a rose or a smoky bottle containing a cobra bobbing in eerie yellow liquid—you just can't quite process it. You have to say "No, no, no, thank you" and step away. Only later can you comprehend the girls' sweet and acrid smell, the sight of their shiny jet hair in the sun, the raking feeling produced by their imploring eyes and claw- ing fingers, somewhere between your heart and your stomach. HIV is like that, too. Sometimes a healthy perspective is all that's needed to be able to see it for what it really is.

CHAPTER
twenty-two

I arrived in Sydney—my last stop on the tour—and was met by the magazine's owner, his wife and others from *POZ* for my second International AIDS Conference.

Everyone was eager to hear how the trip had gone.

Over a dinner of a huge slab of raw Aussie beef, I said, "I think it was a success. They have so many problems preventing and treating infections, especially among the sex workers and IV drug–using communities. One issue is that because the information about the medicine is in English, some of the local doctors don't know how to prescribe it. As a result, people are taking it incorrectly."

"And get this," I said to Tim Horn, the president of AIDS-meds, a company that *POZ*'s parent company had bought the year before I was hired, "there are still people in Taiwan who think you can get HIV from a mosquito."

"No!" Tim said.

"Yes! I had to bring a doctor in to back me up! And no one was going to come to work the day I was scheduled to appear until they brought in a medical expert."

"That's unbelievable!" said Tim.

Tim is one of the foremost experts on AIDS treatment in America, and he is also openly HIV-positive. It was so great to be back around my peers; I hadn't realized how stressful it was to be the only person living with HIV in the midst of a lot of folks who knew nothing about the disease.

A few nights later, Tim and I had dinner in Sydney with Peter Staley, Tim's old boss and the founder of AIDSmeds. Peter was one of the original members of ACT UP—a formidable, Black-Panther-esque group of AIDS activists who did things like chain themselves to the White House gates, solder themselves into pharmaceutical executive offices and, with Sean Strub, POZ's founder, slip a giant condom over Senator Jesse Helms's house. As a member of the new guard, I envied the fervor of those early days, wishing I'd been up on that roof with Sean and Peter.

Peter asked what it was like to deal with the officials on my trip.

"Well, when I left the cocktail party that the American ambassador to Vietnam gave me at his lovely home in Hanoi, I pulled him aside and said he had to get behind clean needle exchange and allow substitution therapy to be introduced to the IV drug–using community in Vietnam. I told him that it was really hard for Vietnamese sex workers to convince the Western business-men and politicos who used their services to use a condom when the men were willing and able to pay five times the going rate to have unprotected sex. I suggested politely that the ambassador help launch an HIV prevention campaign directed at the tourists and businessmen who came to this beautiful country for . . . lei-sure . . . and leaving with more than a fond memory."

Peter said, "Atta girl."

*   *   *

When I returned from the Pacific Rim, it had been a year and a half since I'd started at *POZ*. I was totally exhausted. I still loved my job and all the amazing, inspiring people I met every day through my work, but it's not easy to always be the bearer of bad news, over and over reminding people who thought they were safe from AIDS that they must keep thinking about a subject we'd all like to put out of our minds forever. How, I wondered, had all the activists who'd been doing this work since the early '80s, kept at it?

The first week back from the trip to Asia was hell. I woke up every night at two AM, starving. I'd lie wide awake, staring out the window, waiting for dawn. At the first sign of light, I'd crawl out of my bed and into my clothes, and head for the local diner.

Deprivation creates appreciation. After nearly a month of sitting in front of plates of hacked chicken in garlic, pig's knuckles and Flintstone-sized slabs of Aussie beef, I was delighted to see my toast, jam, bacon and hash browns appear. And yet, nothing tasted the same as it had before my trip; it all tasted artificial. American food offered comfort in its familiarity, but my eyes, mind and palate had been pried wide open by seeing and eating in far-flung places; on a culinary level and beyond, I was no longer convinced that the American way was the right way, let alone the best way, to eat or live.

In Asia, I saw that sharing my story had the power to draw other people out of their silence and pain. But the notion of dedicating my life to leading people down this path was also daunting. For one thing, I worried that if I inspired others to come forward about their HIV status, they wouldn't get the same love and support I had. Luckily, I can say I haven't had one person anywhere in the world ever tell me they regretted breaking their silence about living with HIV. Disclosure is not always pretty and it takes some people a while to come to a place of compassion or comfort, but usually they come around. If they don't, then sometimes it's better for the person to be out of your life. That said, we have a long way to go to protect the human rights of people living with HIV in places like Syria, where the government endorses stoning people living with HIV; Jamaica, where HIV-positive people are stabbed and dragged through the streets; or Egypt, where people living with HIV have been chained to beds and left to die.

After almost a month on the road spending all of my waking hours in intensely emotional situations with people I didn't know, eating food whose names I couldn't pronounce and dealing with climates and pollution levels that were far beyond anything I could ever have imagined, it was so comforting to be home with my family and friends.

While I was grateful for all I'd seen on my voyage, I had a new appreciation for my morning calls to my mom, my dad and my sister, and for doing simple, conquerable things like getting more carrots for the horses and picking up my dry cleaning. I'd spent nearly a month wrestling with questions such as whether the millions of dollars' worth of antiretroviral medications the United States ships abroad would make any difference in a country of starving people with little access to the food and clean water they needed to take, and to stomach, those medications. That is, provided they can travel twenty kilometers barefoot through the leech-infested rice paddies to get to the clinic to get their meds.

Over sushi, shortly after my trip, Susie said, "Tell us about Vietnam!"

The other girls sat around the table waiting raptly. Part of me wanted to tell them about a day trip I took on an antique boat across the sapphire blue Ha Long Bay through the magic mountains rising from the sea. But a bigger part of me wanted them to know about the pain I'd seen. So I said, "I wish you could have seen the faces of the children in the orphanages in Taiwan. One little one, named Benny, looked at me with an expression that revealed that somehow—though he was too young to sit up, or talk—he knew he had been abandoned by parents taken away by AIDS. It felt as if he knew he was considered untouchable. His eyes didn't even follow mine because so few people had ever held him, or looked him in the eye."

The wine was passed around the table.

I wanted to tell them so much more, but I found it nearly impossible to describe what you feel when talking to a woman who sells her body for sex each night to be able to feed her toddlers—when she says, in response to your question about why she doesn't use a condom: "I can have sex with one strange man without a condom and make the same amount as I would if I used a condom and had sex with five men. It takes less time and takes away from my soul less." How can you explain what it feels like to be on a live radio show in Sydney, Australia, and have a caller ask if you don't think you deserve to die for the immoral behavior that led to your getting HIV?

The questions that my trip often raised about AIDS care in America weren't any easier to answer. Why doesn't the government automatically reauthorize the Ryan White CARE Act (a program that gives funding for people who can't afford HIV care)? Why is domestic AIDS funding being slashed? Why can't we develop prevention campaigns that work? Why won't we teach comprehensive sex education or create needle exchange programs when endless scientific studies prove that they work? How do we overcome AIDS apathy? What do we have to do to get the American media to do more—and more positive—stories about people living with HIV stateside? Will we find a cure? Are we even looking in the right places?

So instead, I filled my glass of wine and told them about eating pig's knuckles in the night markets and about the koala bears in the Sydney zoo.

Sensing that I was glossing over the horror, Susie pushed me, "Did your trip make you think we can stop AIDS?"

"I'm not sure. But if there is an answer, I know that it lies in the community itself. The solution to stopping the global spread of AIDS is hidden in the stories of the people living with the virus. In that community, we have a sizable army of untapped force. If people living with HIV are willing to show their faces, that's the best way to convince people that AIDS is still an issue and that it can happen to them."

And my friends looked at my face and nodded.

CHAPTER
twenty-three

Twelve years after I was told I had a year to live, I was reminded that death was a very real possibility.

I went to dinner with my friend Jane one night, and halfway through our meal, my leg began to swell and throb with excruciating pain. I managed to drive home but had to call her within an hour and ask her to come back and take me to the hospital. Jane took me to my local emergency room and sat beside me as I answered questions and filled out paperwork in front of the admitting nurse. As I answered the questions, Jane rubbed my arm. She seemed alarmed; she had never seen me complain, or be ill.

There was no reason to feel hesitant sharing my medical data, even about HIV, in front of Jane. She'd known for almost two years that I was HIV-positive and she was one of my closest and most trusted confidantes. And yet, when the nurse asked, "What drugs are you taking? What was your last CD4 count? And what is your viral load?" I hesitated. Jane and I had always talked about HIV in the abstract. Naming my medications and sharing the specific numbers that spelled out the relative strength of my immune system made HIV real in a way that made Jane raise her eyebrows.

She was one of the first people I told when I was thinking about whether or not to take the job at *POZ*. Sitting in her apartment one winter afternoon almost three years before, I'd said, "I've been offered the editor-in-chief position at an AIDS magazine." I did not tell her I was HIV-positive.

She said, "That's great."

I asked whether she thought it was weird that I would work at a magazine for people with HIV.

And she said, "Why?"

And that was all I needed to know. But though she seemed nonplussed, I still didn't tell her then that I had HIV.

That night in the ER, the on-call doctor came in to examine me; when she poked my knee with her pen, I almost leapt off the exam table in pain.

"Well," she said flatly, "you have a septic knee."

She looked at my chart.

"It's probably gonorrhea," she said.

"What!?" I said, horrified.

"Often, septic joints in young people are associated with gonorrhea," she said.

Well, at least she thought I was young.

Jane's eyes widened, then she looked at the floor. I squirmed under my blanket.

"Could it be anything else?" I asked.

"I suppose so," the doctor said. "I see here," she tapped the chart accusingly with her pen, "that you have HIV."

Now I got it. Because I had one STD, I was a whore and probably had other sexually transmitted diseases.

"I haven't had sex in months. If I'd gotten gonorrhea, wouldn't I have known sooner?" I asked.

She just stared at me.

"I always have protected sex, since I have HIV," I said with a little tremor in my voice.

"Don't worry, it's curable," she said.

"The HIV?" I asked, incredulous. If she thought that, we were out of there.

"No, the septic joint."

I remembered a staph infection I'd gotten at age nineteen when a horse reared up and the chain shank of its lead rope cut open my face. My knee felt as hot and tight as my face had; both times, my body had reacted quickly. I asked, "Could it be staph?"

"It could. But I doubt it. We'll culture it and see."

Then she put on four pairs of gloves, snapping each additional pair on with a defiance that made me want to smack her, and then she drove a six-inch needle under my kneecap. Thankfully, I was holding on to Jane's hand for dear life. The pain was so bad I nearly broke Jane's fingers when I squeezed them.

The nurse gave me an IV of antibiotics and gave Jane a pillow and a blanket so she could stretch out beside me on three hard plastic chairs.

We lay side by side for hours, waiting for a culture result.

In the half-light, I wondered if she believed me, or the doctor. And if she thought I had another STD, how that would affect her opinion of me? Mostly, I didn't want her to think I'd had unprotected sex, as I hadn't. I knew she wanted to leave, both to avoid the discomfort of the chairs, and the tension between the judgmental doctor and me.

But she stayed, and eventually, when the IV antibiotics were finished and I was released from the hospital, she drove me home, helped me fill my prescriptions for more antibiotics and helped me upstairs to my bed.

*   *   *

In the last year, I had switched doctors one more time to Dr. Bauman, who, in addition to being an amazing AIDS doctor, had become an amazing good friend. I called his cell phone and told him what had happened and how I was still in a lot of pain and the swelling wasn't going down.

"I want you to go immediately to a different emergency room," he said in a voice that was so stern, I felt a little wave of fear. "I'm going to call them and tell them how I want them to handle this."

And so, twenty-four hours after my knee first blew up, I was back in the emergency room. They admitted me and hooked me up to several IVs, per Dr. Bauman's instructions.

The antibiotics they'd prescribed at the first hospital were not strong enough; they had had little effect on what was now a raging staph infection and possibly a case of drug-resistant staph, or MRSA, which could be deadly.

My mom joined me in the ER. She looked at me with more concern than I had ever seen directed at me. I did look pretty awful. I hadn't eaten in twenty-four hours and the pain had drawn my face up into a grimace.

She stayed while they drew more blood and admitted me; I was going to have to stay—at least overnight, they said.

Ending up flat on your back without warning, wondering whether you'll ever stand up and walk out of the hospital certainly makes you reflective. My first morning in the hospital, a volunteer came into my room and asked whether I wanted the services of a chaplain. I looked at the nurse and said, "I am going to make it out of here, right?" And she nodded, but not emphatically enough to offer any real comfort. She explained it was standard operating procedure; everyone was offered a visit from the chaplain. I explained that I was studying Buddhism though I had been raised Irish Roman Catholic.

At that, she brightened considerably and said, "Well, in that case, I can give you a rosary. Would you like pink, or black?"

"Pink, please." I wondered who would want a black rosary.

If nothing else, the rosary could double as Zen prayer beads. They were already blessed, she reassured me.

When my dad called and asked if he should fly home to be with me, I got really worried. God, had I survived HIV all these years only to be taken down by staph? Ironically, I had likely gotten the staph when being scratched while trying to rescue some wild cats. I thought about how ironic it would be to die of cat scratch disease after all.

They described the drug cocktail they were shooting into my veins as a bazooka. "Bring it on, *Guns of Navarone* style," I said through a morphine haze to the nurse the first time they connected a clear bag of Zancomycin to my forearm. Another twenty-four hours later, when the medicine had blown out my vein and filled the area under the skin of my forearm, I wasn't laughing. I was terrified and screaming in pain. Somehow, the IV hookup had been botched and the antibiotic was flowing not into my veins as it should have but rather under my skin.

They had moved me to my own room at the end of the hall. At first, I thought my mother had used some of her connections (she used to do fund-raising for our local hospital) to get me a bigger room with a nicer view. But when I kept pressing the nurse's call button and it took an hour for someone to show up, I began to wonder whether I'd been moved to the end of the hall because people were scared to come into my room or to touch me. And because I'd been screaming in pain for the better part of the last two days.

To test the theory, I pressed and pressed the button. After two hours, when no one showed up, I dragged myself out of bed, up onto my crutches and somehow managed to wheel my IVs with me to the door of my room. I yelled down the hall, "Hello? Hello?"

Finally, a nurse came and stood ten feet down the hallway. I asked her for some more toilet paper. She disappeared for a moment; by the time she returned, I was sitting on the edge of my bed shaking with pain. From the doorway, she tossed the roll onto the bed beside me and walked away.

I was so shocked, I said nothing. I just struggled back to my feet and hobbled to the bathroom. I never knew whether it was the HIV or the staph that made her afraid to come into my room—but either way, you'd think a hospital nurse would have handled it better.

As I lay back on my bed, forlorn, I remembered a study that amfAR (Foundation for AIDS Research) had commissioned among a large sample of Americans. The results were terrifying: nearly 60 percent of Americans said they would be "somewhat or not at all comfortable with an HIV-positive woman providing them with childcare"; nearly 50 percent said they would be "somewhat or not at all comfortable with an HIV-positive woman serving them in a restaurant" and 26 percent said they would be "somewhat or not at all comfortable working closely with an HIV-positive woman." Ninety percent of Americans said they would be "somewhat or not at all comfortable dating someone who is HIV-positive"; 92 percent said the same of marrying someone living with HIV and one in five Americans said they would not be comfortable with having an HIV-positive woman as a close friend.

It wasn't just my imagination that people with HIV were stigmatized; we had empirical, scientific data that confirmed our worst nightmare.

Hospitals are like casinos. When you're in them, you have no awareness of the passage of time, the changing weather or what's happening in the outside world. You end up watching old Judy Garland movies and feeling lobotomized by countless hours of daytime soaps and Rachael Ray. The only hint that the external world still existed came one evening when a string of ambulances, fire trucks and marching bands passed along the street beside my seventh-story hospital window. I heard the blaring sirens and beating drums faintly through the seemingly hurricane-proof glass windows that are sealed shut, presumably so you don't hurl yourself out in despair—something I considered doing when the nutritionist denied me my breakfast order of bananas, ice cream and chocolate sauce. She suggested I try the oatmeal instead.

I also heard the unmistakable tinkling of the Good Humor truck. I wondered whether I could get past the nurses' station, downstairs in the elevator and across the street on crutches before he got away. I would have killed someone for a butterscotch sundae. But I could only press my nose against the cool glass and watch summer pass me by.

Not many people came to see me. But those who did looked so scared that I hoped no one else would come. When I broke my ankle a few years ago, people were amazing; they finally had a visible concrete reason to offer condolences and send flowers. They also knew I was going to get better. So they visited, all smiles and gifts and jokes.

But the severity of the staph infection (and perhaps fear that they might catch it) kept most people at bay. For me at least, it was actually refreshing in a twisted sort of way to have a real reason for people to fear me physically.

My mother, of course, came and sat by my bed. In the beginning of the week, when my temperature hovered around 105 and my body was not responding to the medicines, I could tell she was frightened. We both were. Strangely, after all the years we'd thought about, talked about, and even joked about death, when it seemed as if it could actually come, we both fell silent. I could tell how scared she was because she didn't bring her usual cheer-kit of Pecan Sandies, gossip magazines and funny cards. Instead, she brought some cans of Ensure, because I was basically starving to death, and nervously rearranged the bouquets of flowers that were so numerous it looked as if I had already died. It was eerie to be surrounded by so many brightly colored blooms and still be able to see them myself.

Tracy and my dad called constantly; Tracy, as she always is, was impervious to fear. There wasn't the slightest hint of it in her voice. She ribbed me for watching terrible TV and let me know throughout the day that she was going to yoga, shopping for food with her son, meeting Josh for dinner, anything she could do to give me something to think about. My dad was concerned to see that I was getting the right medical care and asked to call my doctor and talk to him himself. I laughed—once a CEO, always a CEO. It wasn't that he didn't trust my opinion of my doctor's expertise; it was just that he wanted to manage something to feel that he could help influence the outcome of my sickness. He offered to fly east to see me.

Several of my family's friends also came by; but again, seeing the concern on their faces terrified me. So I asked my mom to tell people that I was too weak to have visitors. And to please bring me some butterscotch, which, god bless her, she did.

Finally, the new drugs started working and I had surgery on my knee to clean out the infection. Though I was still in pain, incapacitated and weak, I began to feel that I would make it out alive.

After not washing my hair for five days (I know, gross) and then washing it with whatever the hospital gave me and being unable to brush it or dry it (they only gave me one of those tiny men's combs and a thin scratchy towel the size of a Kleenex) I fell asleep on it for hours in a painkiller fog. The next morning when the nurse came in, I sat up in bed and seeing my mile-high mop, she said, "Oh, you did your hair!" And she was totally serious. Only in New Jersey would someone think I had styled my hair to look like it did.

I was just glad to be awake whatever state I was in.

The day I got to leave the hospital, I was afraid. It seemed as if I'd been in the hospital for a month (it had been a week). I felt that I'd forgotten how to eat, walk, sleep, even converse.

Despite my fears that the infection was linked to the HIV, my doctors reassured me repeatedly that the staph infection was neither related to nor made worse by HIV. It was simply a bacteria that could be controlled with the help of the right antibiotic. It was simply a reminder that HIV was not the only thing I had to worry about. It was also reassuring to know that my HIV-challenged body could take a wallop like that and rebound.

The morning I was scheduled to leave the hospital, as I was joyously packing, I realized I hadn't allowed myself until that very moment the thought that I'd definitely be going home. When my temperature soared to 105 and the painkillers were no longer working and we weren't sure exactly what we were dealing with nor whether the antibiotic regimen was effective, there were times that a dark corner of my mind entertained the thought that I might need the chaplain's services after all.

There were two full days that I can't remember clearly. I remember feeling as if my whole body was on fire, then suddenly, that it was icy cold. My head felt as if it was slowly swelling until it would pop and my leg felt like it was trapped under a burning building. I vaguely recall grabbing the arm of the night nurse and screaming, "I am in a developed nation, on morphine and antibiotics—how the hell can I feel this bad? You HAVE to help me, please . . ."

To distract myself from the pain, I stared at the TV, trying to find the most ridiculous shows to make myself laugh—something I did like a crazy person through a whole hour of Hip Hop Abs. At some point, my laughter turned to sobs and then, in the middle of the second night, I slid into that protective place where the nerves, having been on overload for so many hours, just stopped feeling, and my body was blissfully numb. With my thoughts gone totally awry, I struggled to focus on anything in the world beyond my mind, just to prove to myself that I was still on the planet. I remember seeing the nurse's name written in a giant chicken scrawl on the erasable board by the door, and I repeated over and over to myself: Sandra, Sandra, Sandra . . .

To suddenly find myself hooked up to machines writhing in pain despite morphine, not caring what day it was or even whether it was day or night was a real shocker. As I waited for the cultures of my blood to grow whatever brand of bug had infected me, I got a tiny sense of the terror that those in the early days of the AIDS epidemic experienced, and that far too many people today know—the notion that either the doctors don't know what's wrong with you—or they do, but they don't know how, or don't have the tools, to cure what ails you.

In the elevator on the way out of the hospital, I was sitting slumped in my wheelchair across from an elderly Asian man.

A hospital worker said cheerfully, "Going home today, are we?"

Both the man and I nodded. Our eyes met and he smiled at me. Then he laughed. And I laughed back. I knew exactly how he was feeling—neither of us could believe we were going home. They wheeled us out onto the sidewalk and I took my first breath of fresh air in a week and felt the sun soak into my face. Our families went to get the cars, leaving the old man and me sitting side by side breathing in unison. I closed my eyes and felt his spindly hand rest on my forearm, which was bruised and swollen from the multiple IVs. He squeezed it lightly.

We never said a word to each other but as he drove away, he turned and looked out of the back window of his family's car. We said a whole lot more with our silent understanding than we could have with words.

When I got home, after sleeping for a couple of days and having successfully learned to use the IV port in my arm (they'd sewn a PIC line into my bicep so that a catheter could run through my vein down into my heart), I realized that not since I was diagnosed with HIV had I savored life so much. Every brush with death has a way of recalibrating our dials so we remember what's truly important. Embracing mortality has a funny way of reminding us to appreciate life. My first bite of ice cream at home was amazing—and perhaps because my leg was still recovering from surgery, and I was on crutches, I walked a whole lot slower, which afforded me the time to smell the wild roses and freshly cut grass as I cruised slowly up the driveway listening to the crickets and the owls on the farm.

I called Jane to tell her I was home, that I was okay—and that I didn't have gonorrhea. She was relieved, as I was, on all counts.

CHAPTER
twenty-four

I was scheduled to go to Africa with the Elizabeth Glaser Pediatric AIDS Foundation (EGPAF) in July, just after I was released from the hospital. I struggled with whether or not it made sense for me to go, given that I'd just recovered from a massive, systemic bacterial infection. And I was supposed to go to Nairobi, where, because of political unrest, American diplomats had recently been pulled out. Between disease and the dangers of being an American amid international political strife it probably would have been rational to stay home. But as I had believed from the earliest days, part of the secret to my survival was not thinking or acting as if I was immune compromised. With all due respect to my mortality, I didn't want to live in fear. And in order to truly be qualified to write about HIV, I felt as if I needed to experience AIDS in Africa firsthand.

My mom and dad asked me to reconsider. But after calling friends in the State Department and speaking with people at EGPAF, I decided that it was worth the reasonable risk. We were traveling to ensure that the PEPFAR funds that the Bush

Administration had given to Kenya and South Africa were being put to proper use through EGPAF's programs, which focus mainly on preventing mother-to-child transmission of HIV in the developing world. Since we were part of a group of people who were trying to save their women and children, I doubted that anyone in either country was really going to try to hurt us. So after getting inoculated, I packed my bags and was off to Nairobi, Kenya.

I knew from my trip to the Far East that a lot of things about living with HIV are universal. But Africa taught me that where people live with HIV has everything to do with whether they will live or die.

Nothing I could have ever imagined could have prepared me for seeing people trying to survive AIDS in rural East Africa or in the slums outside Johannesburg. Several months prior to my trip, I had asked Pam Barnes, then the CEO of EGPAF, to take me with her to see the foundation's work in the field. She said it would not be glamorous, that she was going to Kenya and South Africa to make the rounds of clinics and other recipients of their support. She said people would be sick and the conditions would be rustic. I told her I wanted to see reality—whatever that was.

We met in the Nairobi airport in August. Pam is a lovely, gracious, petite brunette with the manners and sensibilities of a seasoned diplomat and the determination and ferocity of a pit bull. She picked me up at the Nairobi airport with her support staff and we drove directly to our hotel. Nairobi was intensely dangerous. I could feel eyes all over me even as I was walking down the hallway to my room in the supposed safety of our hotel.

The next day, we started making the rounds of AIDS clinics scattered all over the eastern and western provinces of Kenya to see whether the drugs and information that EGPAF provided were succeeding in preventing mother-to-child transmission of HIV.

Named after Elizabeth Glaser, who was married to Paul Michael Glaser (Starsky of *Starsky and Hutch*), the foundation continued Elizabeth's legacy of advocating on behalf of children with HIV, and working to create a generation free of HIV. Elizabeth had two children; both were born with HIV because she wasn't aware she had the disease until her youngest child was diagnosed with HIV. She dedicated her life to trying to save the lives of her own children—and all others around the world. Her daughter, Ariel, succumbed to the disease, but her son, Jake, lived. EGPAF's mission seems achievable. By administering antiretroviral medication to HIV-positive mothers and giving their babies a course of the drugs after they are born EGPAF has had nearly a 100 percent efficacy rate for prevention.

The first pediatric clinic we visited was in a small Kenyan village. It was a low, sprawling cement building with no doors or windows, full of young mothers with children in various stages of distress. A few held children on their hips, those with tuberculosis sputtered and coughed, others sweated with malarial fevers. All of the women were dressed in their Sunday best; bright swirls of colorful fabric wrapped their pregnant but somehow still tiny bodies, as bottles of wine might be wrapped at the holidays in festive paper. Many of the children lay wide-eyed in disbelief at their pain in their mothers' arms; some were lethargic, others suffered more actively. The scene reminded me of the waiting room at my first doctor's office nearly eleven years ago. I pinched the inside of my arm to keep from crying.

Peter, the country director for EGPAF in Kenya, led us

through the clinic with the doctors and nurses. The doctors told us how the funding and medicines EGPAF provided had saved hundreds of lives in the last year.

"Will these kids make it?" I asked one doctor, pointing to the sea of sick children sprawled around the room on low beds and iron cribs.

"Yes, thankfully, most of them will be fine," he reassured me. "They got here, that is often the hard part."

It was the only clinic in the extended surrounding area that had access to the life-saving AIDS medicines, and thankfully, the word that EGPAF had the answer to having an HIV-free baby had gotten around; the local young women walked, sometimes as far as fifteen or twenty kilometers, sometimes after their water had broken, to get there. Other than trying to prevent their babies from becoming HIV-positive, there was no incentive for these women to give birth at a clinic as opposed to staying home. At home, they had privacy, food and the support of people they knew. The teenage girls who had come alone to a place with no privacy, no food and no familiar faces did so because they understood that their children didn't have to carry the virus even if they themselves did.

The midwives, working three to four to a clinic, often handled as many as twenty to thirty births a day. Many times, they would find themselves counseling women who were well along in labor, to try to get the mother-to-be to agree to be tested for HIV. Then they would test them, give the woman their diagnosis, again, mid-labor, and if necessary convince them to take their first dose of antiretroviral medications hours before they welcomed their child into the world.

The idea that HIV could be prevented was new to these young women. Because the stigma surrounding HIV was so debilitating—should a young woman test positive, her husband would

often disown her, throwing her out of their home and their village even though he had likely cheated and given it to her—that
people didn't want to get tested for HIV. But some primal mother
instinct kicked in with these young women, making them willing,
at the eleventh hour, to face that which they were terrified of to
save their own child.

There were three sections to the hospital: one for women
who were in labor, the delivery area, and the recovery room.
As I walked through a door labeled "Theater," which is what
they called the delivery room, I was hit by a smell so intense
I almost went down on my knees. In the square cement box
were four green rubber beds on gurneys, each positioned above
a drain in the floor so the bed could be hosed down before the
next delivery. The midwives were especially proud of their new
"curtains." They had finally gotten the money, and supplies,
to hang a cross of pipes between the four beds so they could
drape sheets on them, offering the women at least a suggestion
of privacy.

I walked back out into the hallway to join the group.

"How do the women get home?" I asked as we looked through
a glass window into a room where the young mothers slept curled
around babies so tiny they were barely visible.

"They walk, just like they did to get here," a nurse said.

The hospital had no pillows, no blankets, no food, no painkillers and not enough room; the women were allowed to rest for
a time after delivery, then they had to get up and go—to make
room for the next young girl trying to bring a healthy baby into
the world.

We left the clinic and drove several hours over dirt roads
with potholes so deep that the truck had several spare tires—
just in case. We passed miles and miles of pineapple farms and
coffee plantations; men and boys walked or rode bicycles along

the roadside, many of them wearing rumpled dusty suits, and no shoes.

At the second clinic, we walked in through the intake area. Several young women sat in various degrees of pain as they waited to go into delivery

One young woman, wearing a brightly striped shirt on top and an orange towel on the lower half of her body, was bent over her knees and rocking back and forth. Occasionally, she caught my eye, and looked down at the floor when the contractions came. It seemed awkward for us to be standing there, listening to a lecture on the history and efficacy of the hospital's pediatric AIDS program while the young women around us got progressively deeper into labor. Hoping to distract the girl in the orange towel from her pain, and wanting them to understand that we came in peace to help, I asked the nurse to tell her why we were there and that I too had HIV.

The nurse sat beside the young girl, talking rapidly in Swahili. While she spoke, the girl stopped her rocking and, sitting up straight, stared at me. We smiled at each other. I pointed to the chair next to her and she nodded. As I sat down, a contraction bent her in two again. Gingerly, I laid a hand on the small of her back and rubbed it in small circles. She looked at me with her head turned sideways, laying her cheek on her forearms, which were folded on her knees. In between grimaces, she smiled and I kept rubbing.

We left the clinic around eleven and returned in the afternoon. When we came back, my new friend in the orange towel had delivered a gorgeous little boy. His crazy tuft of downy hair reminded me of that on top of Benny's head—the little boy who stole my heart at the orphanage in Taiwan. For a second, my memories of all the children I'd seen affected by HIV blended together; the newborns here in Kenya sipping mouthfuls of liquid AZT; the babies lying catatonic in cribs in Taipei who never needed medications, as they had been born HIV-free but were still being thrown away simply because they had emerged from the body of an HIV-positive parent; and small kids selling fans and roses on the streets of Vietnam while their HIV-positive mothers worked the docks to try to make enough money to feed the family.

In a way, the Kenyan baby, wrapped in a candy-colored fleece and clutched closely to his mother's chest, was so much luckier than his orphan cousins halfway across the world—especially if he was given proper medication and eventually tested HIV-negative, which he was likely to do. This boy was still with his mother. The sad thing to me, as I absorbed the joy and beauty of his mother's face, was that her odds of seeing her boy grow up were still not great. There was no guarantee that she'd be able to access the medications she'd need to survive. Or that her country's government would be able to afford giving them to her for as long as she needed them.

I thought of my own mother and father, and how torturous it must be for them to know that there isn't much more they can do than all the incredible things they have already done for me to keep me alive. I also thought of Tracy, and her three-year-old son, and her second baby now growing inside her. Because we lived so far away from each other, I had missed watching most of her mothering. But on the few occasions that I had the privilege of seeing her handle her son, I saw such love and tenderness— and that too seemed a universal truth: put a baby in the hands of its mother and all the pain that it caused coming into the world—and after it emerged—vanishes. And tell a mother that her child is in danger of dying and she will do anything to save it—even walk twenty kilometers, through the bush, barefoot, in labor.

While it was encouraging to see the progress being made with

EGPAF's help, I couldn't help thinking how none of this had to be. If only Thabo Mbeki, the former South African president, had not supported the "denialists," who claimed that AIDS was not caused by HIV but was merely a "syndrome" arising from poverty and malnutrition. There is still much misinformation, because of his position, around AIDS in Africa.

About a week later, after spending many fourteen hour days in clinics in Kenya and then South Africa, I needed a break from the harsh realities of AIDS in Africa.

Back in Nairobi, over dinner at the hotel, I downed multiple glasses of South African wine, trying to eliminate the cries of the newborns from my head.

During dinner, a bottle of wine had been sent to our table by a group of men sitting nearby. When it happened, I hadn't paid much attention, as I figured one of the ten people I was dining with knew someone in the restaurant. But as we finished dessert, a crew of gorgeous guys walked by our table—they had joked with us in French as we'd checked into the hotel several days before. One of them, a tall dirty-blond-haired man with piercing eyes stopped, pointed at me and said something I did not understand, in French. Pam laughed and said, "He said the wine was for you." The table raised their glasses and I turned the same color red as the viscous liquid sliding down the crystal.

On the way out of the restaurant, I passed the hotel bar and noticed the Frenchmen sitting inside. I excused myself to say good night and to thank them for the wine.

Several hours later, we'd turned the staid, Masterpiece-Theatre-esque hotel bar into a thumping disco. We flipped between African music videos and coverage of the summer Olympics on the plasma TV and were joined by a flight crew from Malaysia Air. Soon the lights got lower, the coffee tables became dance platforms and someone turned the music up so loud that we had to use sign language to communicate. After all the tension of being in the clinics with the sick children it seemed strange to feel like dancing, but somehow, it was just what the doctor ordered.

As light crept in through the windows, I glanced anxiously at my watch and Franky, the Frenchman who had masterminded the wine move, asked if he could walk me to my room.

En route, we passed Pam, who was on her way to the gym. She waved at me with a mischievous grin and said she'd see me at breakfast—in half an hour.

Franky and I paused outside my door. As he leaned in to kiss me, I realized that he had no idea why I was in South Africa, or that I was living with HIV. Putting a hand firmly on the muscles of his chest, which had become defined by hours of kite-sailing all over the world, I said, "Franky, I have to tell you, I have HIV."

"*Le sida?*" he said in French. Their acronym for AIDS.

"*Oui.*"

"*Pas de mal,*" he said, leaning in.

For a split second I had remembered what it was like to have HIV not be a barrier between a man and me.

I thanked him for the wine—and the dancing—and went inside to shower and dress in preparation for another day in the field.

That day, the last of our trip, we went into a remote rural village to see the impact of another program on a community fighting HIV. As soon as we parked on the dirt road, a crowd of men, women children gathered around the van. Even in that remote area people were getting access to antiretroviral drugs and being

successfully encouraged to get tested and treated and adhere to
their treatments.

We walked into a simple concrete and corrugated steel structure and the sound of hundreds of people singing raised high
the rafters. From the table they had set for us at the front of the
room, I watched the women dance, the men wave their arms
above their heads and the kids giggle. After the singing stopped,
Pam gave a lovely speech and said she hoped that more people
would come forward to get care. People cheered and danced some
more. Several of the children gave testimonies and thanks and at
the end, they showed us a lavish spread of gifts they had brought
for us. There were wooden trays filled with handmade crafts and
amazing vegetables. A little boy dragged me to an overturned
basket. He pointed at it. I lifted it up and found a cluster of baby
rabbits.

"He wants you to have them," my translator said.

I looked at the small child whose clothes were so thin I could
see his belly button through his T-shirt. His face was hollowed by
all the food he'd not eaten.

"Please thank him for me," I said. "But tell him I can't possibly take them."

She paused, then relayed what I said to the boy.

He looked crestfallen.

She explained, "He thinks you are disappointed with his
gift."

"Oh!" I said. "Please tell him it is the nicest and most generous gift I've been given but the authorities won't let me take
them on the plane, so he must hold my gift here for me and take
care of them himself."

She told the boy what I said and his dark face split wide in a
flash of white teeth.

Another man dragged me to a display he'd made of a newspaper article that told his story about how he'd come forth, unafraid, to tell his community that he was HIV-positive. He'd become a local hero. He had a posse of young men around him who stared at me and nodded emphatically while the man spoke to me in his native tongue.

I looked at my translator. "Please tell him," I said, "that I think he is very brave and that his bravery will save lives."

She did, and after listening to her words, the tall, skinny, deeply black man extended his arms and hugged me hard against his tall, hard, thinly muscled frame.

We left the village carrying armfuls of handmade crafts. I wished I had known they would be giving us presents, as I would have brought something for them. But the translators explained that all the things we were given were in response to what the United States had already doled out in the form of drugs, money for clinics and money for medical staff.

As we drove away in a cloud of red South African dust, the little boy I'd met ran alongside the truck clutching a tiny puff of a rabbit, in his fingers holding it up in the air for me to see.

I slept on the floor of the plane while traveling home from South Africa to New York by way of Amsterdam. I woke only once, when the plane bucked and shuddered as we skirted a massive electrical storm over the Sahara. Sitting up in a sleepy daze, I watched bolts of light finger across the sky and thought the tumult and miles-high pile of clouds looked like two worlds colliding. Indeed, in my life, they had.

CHAPTER

twenty-five

Africa was the final piece of a puzzle I'd been trying to put together for years in my head. It convinced me that the answer to stopping the devastation caused by AIDS lies in the destigmatization of AIDS and the subsequent ability of the community of people living with HIV to come forward to each other, and to the wide world. The trip to Africa removed the last shreds of hesitation I had when telling people about my disease. Which is why I barely paused before answering when Keith asked me why I was an AIDS activist.

I'd met Keith earlier in the summer, while I was recovering from the staph infection and before I went to Africa. My friends and I had started frequenting a local restaurant in Lambertville where his jazz quartet played on Thursday nights. I had noticed him and several times my friends and I had hung out with his band.

One night, he noticed the large bandage I had on my upper left arm and asked about it. He had merry, playful eyes, and my first instinct was to tell a tall tale about the life-saving portal sewn into my bicep. But his eyes also revealed a depth that made me sense that truth was a currency he'd appreciate. I told him about the staph infection and explained that I was self-administering medicines through a line sewn into my heart to save my life.

I watched his face closely to detect any trace of repulsion. But there was none.

He barely blinked his thick lashes. I was encouraged that my illness did not push him away.

We talked several more times in the group of people who had cocktails together, after his gig. Each time, I was constantly and pleasantly being surprised. He always said just the thing I wanted to hear. He was whip smart, hilariously funny and wildly creative in his thinking.

One night, after he played, I asked Keith if he'd like to have coffee with me sometime—and he asked if I would like to go to have a beer with him that night.

I said, "Sure."

We went to a local bar to listen to live rock music. Some of Jody's good friends, many of whom I hadn't seen since his memorial service, walked by.

One of them, John, had been with Jody in the canoe the night he drowned. He stopped, grabbed my arm and said, "I was at a Super Bowl party and I saw you on TV. It was crazy."

Another said, "Yeah, I saw you too!"

They had seen a public service announcement for AIDS awareness that I did for Viacom. I watched Keith out of the corner of my eye as they talked about it. But he had half an ear on another conversation and, thankfully, wasn't tuned in to what they were saying.

When Keith and I moved from the bar and sat down at a little wooden table by the stage, he asked, "What do you do?"

"I'm an editor and an AIDS activist," I said. "I work for a

magazine called *POZ,* and a website, poz.com, for people living with and affected by HIV/AIDS."

"Why do you do that?" he asked.

I took a big swig of my beer before continuing.

I could tell from the icy feeling along the back of my neck and the dull ache in my gut that I liked Keith way more than I had allowed myself to acknowledge. And then, because I knew I didn't want to spend weeks worrying about how he'd take The News while I got to know him and perhaps fall in love with him, I decided to get it over with, up front. So I said, "I do that because I have HIV."

"Wow," he said. "Tell me about it."

And I did.

He listened intently with a compassionate expression while I told him about my life; how I'd come in contact with the disease, and how I'd tried to do my best to come to terms with living with the virus—while facing the reality that I could still possibly die from it.

I was afraid that so much information given so soon might chase Keith away, but I was no longer able to tolerate people who could not appreciate what and why I did what I did. I had promised myself that I would never again be with someone who was incapable of handling the disease. I deserved to be treated just like anyone else. From my budding feelings I knew I would be devastated if HIV proved a barrier between us and I didn't want to become more emotionally attached if this was the case.

We hung out over the next few weeks, walking across the river from Lambertville, New Jersey, to New Hope, Pennsylvania, to have drinks, dinner or coffee, wandering slowly above the river where I'd lost Jody, under the metal struts of the bridge that was strewn with hundreds of dazzling spiderwebs.

There was both an ease and excitement between us. We spent hours on the phone and spoke of everything—except my disease.

Keith handled the HIV totally in stride. He got tested for HIV of his own volition. He told his friends. The guys in his band. His parents. It was, refreshingly, not a big deal.

Earlier in the year, before Keith and I met, I had been featured in a fashion advertising campaign for Kenneth Cole. In addition to selling his clothes, the campaign was intended, as were many of his ads, to raise awareness for a social cause. In the case of the campaign I appeared in, the idea was that you could be different—and still excel. The theme was non-uniform thinking and the non-traditional models included, in addition to myself, a woman who had had both her lower legs amputated—and rebuilt by engineers at MIT so that she was faster than people with their biological legs; a quadriplegic rugby player; a woman who had fully tattooed both arms and legs; a practicing and turban-wearing Sikh; a lesbian couple who had a child; and a gay Republican. We were all somehow the kind of people who made others uncomfortable, but we had all risen above whatever natural or self-inflicted challenges we had to overcome.

In my case, it was tricky: how do you show that someone is HIV-positive? I talked to the art directors about how we might handle showing my HIV status. The answer came when I was filmed in the accompanying video for the Kenneth Cole website. While being interviewed, I said that when I was first diagnosed, I considered getting a tattoo on my upper arm that said "HIV+." I thought my body could tell people about my HIV status so my lips didn't have to. Back then, I could never have imagined telling everyone I had HIV. I said that after consideration, I decided that getting the tattoo was too fatalistic—I wanted to believe there would be a day when there would no longer be any HIV in the world. On the other hand, even if they cured the disease, I wouldn't mind wearing a badge that forever reminded me of all I'd been through.

I arrived at the Kenneth Cole shoot in downtown Manhattan and was escorted upstairs. I walked through a pair of brushed steel doors into a huge white studio where various teams of people (photo, hair and makeup, wardrobe and client) clustered in their respective corners. The famous photographer Terry Richardson was shooting the campaign.

I went to the wardrobe people first. They picked out a tissue-thin chartreuse shirt and black skirt that hugged my body so tightly, I had to remove all my undergarments. To my great relief, the other half of the outfit was a thick, belted, black trench coat that I wrapped around the transparent dress.

The Kenneth Cole executives gave the instructions to make me up "naturally." As a result, I emerged from makeup looking anemic.

When it was my turn, I stepped in front of Terry's lens.

He walked around me, snapping cautiously.

I was so stiff I could barely crack a smile.

Terry stopped shooting and whispered to the executives.

I panicked. Was I being rejected from the campaign?

The makeup man escorted me back to his chair and within ten minutes, had changed my face completely. Armed now with giant smoky eyes and a glossy red mouth, I was able to preen in front of Terry in a way that made him start pressing the button on his camera.

At first, he shot slowly, deliberately. Then, asking his crew to turn the music up, he came closer, so I could see the different hues that made up the plaid of his flannel shirt. He looked at me over the thick black rims of his science teacher glasses and asked whether I could lift up the shirt.

"Up to where?" I asked, nervously.

"Just so we can see your stomach," he said gently. "Could you, perhaps, take the bottom hem of the shirt and . . . hold it in your teeth?"

They were going to add the "HIV+" tattoo onto my body in post-production; we had discussed two possible places for it, one on my bicep, the other on my lower stomach.

I looked at the executives, who nodded.

"Okay," I said.

And then, Terry started shooting. Fast and furious. And the music kept getting turned up louder and louder and he kept saying, "Yeah, that's it. Just like that. Perfect."

It felt great to be unabashedly sexy.

Months later, after the photo shoot, one morning while I was driving into Manhattan, I got a call from Jennifer, my managing editor and dear friend, who said she'd emerged from the subway in Grand Central and seen my face, four feet high, in front of her on a Kenneth Cole poster.

We met at the office and she walked with me back over to the train station with me so I could see my mug plastered on the side of the Kenneth Cole store.

"Jesus," I said.

"What?" she asked.

"I don't know," I said. "It's just so weird. Three years ago, I was undone by the idea of having my face on *POZ*. And now I have my face in Grand Central station, and I'm actually calm about it."

"Well, maybe that's because you already know how people will react," she said.

And I looked at the mahogany-haired woman whom I had worked beside for the three hardest years of my life and smiled. She knew me so well. She was right. There could be no more fear, because I'd already slain that dragon publicly.

When I agreed to take the job at *POZ*, I underestimated the strength that's required to stand up to stigma every day. It's hard to describe, but even people who know that you're positive, believe that you're a good person anyway, don't fear you physically and admire what you do, glance sideways at you every now and then. Maybe it's just a remnant of incredulity that makes them peer at you strangely when you're not looking. I'm not sure I'm reading it right. Maybe it's pity. Maybe it's fear. All I know is that there are very few people who treat me exactly the same as they did before they knew I was HIV-positive. Many of them are kinder. Some of them are more attentive. Some are more curious about me as a woman. And some have gone away. Some have needed to.

Few people were as mature, kind and accepting about HIV as Keith was. If it was ever a big deal to him, he never let me feel that it was. We barely spoke of the virus.

Instead, we spent nights laughing at random YouTube videos, cooking together, playing music we loved for each other and walking around his neighborhood and the farm where I lived. One Saturday morning, he took me to his local taxidermist, and we watched as they skinned two coyotes strung up on meat hooks by their back legs. That's when I knew we were destined to be together. Who else would understand my fascination with death, or my appreciation of an act that honors the remnants of a body after a spirit has left it by giving it a second life? Few others would be willing, as he was that day, to stand with a scarf over his mouth, breathing in the sickening smell of dead coyotes, for their girlfriends. To me, a mark of real love is the ability to do something that's unpleasant for ourselves if it gives joy to someone we care for.

Unlike with anyone I'd dated before, I felt completely and unapologetically myself with Keith. That was both a testament to who he is, his open-hearted loving and my firm resolution to never again compromise myself in the name of love.

We walked through the end of summer nights under the full moon; he wrote songs for me and I dreamed, and daydreamed, of him. Even as we fell in love, I realized that our connection superseded the limitations of a normal relationship.

One night, not long after we met, I was having dinner with my mother and two of her friends—Pam and Ann—and I asked Keith if he wanted to join us. He said he would and offered to cook the food we'd bought at the farmers' market that morning. I called my mom and asked if she and Pam and Ann wanted to come to my house instead of meeting at a restaurant as we'd planned. She said yes. "Oh, and by the way," I said, "my new boyfriend will be here, too."

When my mom and her friends arrived, Keith was cooking homemade butternut squash soup and I was arranging the oysters. I gave everyone a drink as Keith put the finishing touches on our meal.

Over dinner, we talked about all kinds of things: how my mother had coped for years trying to help me emotionally without being able to tap into the support of her own friends until recently; how everyone, especially Pam and Ann, had made me feel when I finally disclosed to my hometown; how the news of my disclosure had affected them; how it had resulted in their talking to their own children about AIDS; how they themselves had gotten tested; how my mom felt now that everything was out in the open.

During dinner, Keith mostly listened. In a lull in the conversation, while I was clearing plates, Ann asked him, "Keith, what was your experience with HIV before you met Regan?"

Keith, who was twenty-nine at the time, said, "None. Regan is the first person I've personally met who has HIV."

We all were slack-jawed. For those of us who'd seen firsthand how AIDS ravages a body, who'd all known the brave activism on the part of the gay community in the '80s, who'd seen so many people die from AIDS, it was shocking to us that a person could grow up without knowing someone with HIV.

But Keith and much of the rest of his generation had.

As astounding as it was to think that HIV could fail to loom large on someone's radar, it also gave me great hope. To know that my boyfriend, my mother, her friends and I—three different generations—could talk freely about AIDS convinced me that we can profoundly change the world's view of the disease. So that one day, AIDS would be relegated to its rightful place—as just another disease among diseases. Keith's mind had not been tainted by all of the factors that created the enormous stigma around AIDS; to him, it was merely a retrovirus that can cause illness if left untreated.

After my mom and her friends left, Keith asked, "Do you want to hear my new song?"

I said, "Of course."

"It's called 'In an Airfield,'" he said and I smiled in our candle-lit room, remembering the rapture we'd shared among the moon shadows on the same airfield where I'd seen a horse and rider galloping with joy the day that I first moved to the farm.

He pushed PLAY on his recorder and I listened to the lyrics.

"Your wishes and demons have come to see / the meaning of choices I can't make / in an ocean of diamonds with lovers and lives / that I can't take away from you / take away the black of love / daytime is nighttime is love is love is love . . ."

Hearing Keith's lyrics and reflecting on the ease of our love in spite of HIV and his acceptance and openness made me realize that it is absolutely possible to bring this disease out of the darkness—and into the light—so that it can be seen clearly and no longer be feared.

The only thing that makes HIV scary and upsetting is the way we look at it, or, more accurately, how we fail to see it for what it is. Despite society's misperception that HIV is somehow drawn to people of a lesser moral caliber, HIV is nothing more than a brainless retrovirus that couldn't possibly make a judgment call about those it infects. Our ability to overcome it lies in our willingness to see it simply as a disease like any other.

We may not conquer AIDS in my lifetime but we must immediately conquer the stigma surrounding this disease so that we may better prevent people from getting it and that whatever time those of us living with the virus have left on the planet is spent full of as much joy and dignity as possible. Because even people with HIV/AIDS deserve to be loved.

That is what I wanted to tell you.

epilogue

I am not a walking biohazard. I am not a heated container of deadly viral particles. I am not sick. I will not kill you. I refuse to be part of a strange tribe of people, bound by bad biology. I will no longer be misunderstood, deeply feared for the human immunodeficiency virus I carry, bearing a crippling stigma. I am not ashamed. And I am silent no more.

AIDS is a disease—not a crime, nor a punishment, nor a reflection of the moral caliber of the person living with it. HIV is an equal opportunity offender, something that can be survived and something that should be avoided at all costs. It is a retrovirus. It is preventable. It is not shameful. And if you think it can't find you, or the people you love, you are risking lives.

It is something we must tell each other about because HIV threatens to make you sick, but the stigma and silence surrounding HIV/AIDS surely kill.

Won't you please help me spread the word so we can stop the spread of HIV?

For information about getting tested for, treating and preventing HIV, please visit www.poz.com.

Acknowledgments

Thank you to my father, David Hofmann; my mother, Nancy Cosentino, and her late husband, Frank Cosentino; and my sister, Tracy Hofmann Rosen, and her husband, Josh Rosen, for your extraordinary strength, friendship, courage, grace, lightness and love. Thanks to Asher and Harper Rosen, for providing me with added incentive for fighting for a generation free of HIV/AIDS.

Thanks to my extended family—aunts Betty, Gabe, Kay and Kathleen; uncles Harold, Jim, John and Mike; and all my cousins—for your support and love over the years.

A special remembrance to my grandparents: Harold and Mary Hofmann and Frank and Betty Holmes. You flowed through me during the writing of this book.

All of the incredible doctors who have kept me alive and kicking despite HIV.

I also offer deepest gratitude (in alphabetical order) to the following people I cherish:

Ian Anderson, for your leadership at POZ and your kind, savvy counsel.

Peter Arnold, Tim Braun and Bea and Lily, for making life magical.

Pam Barnes, for showing me Africa and for helping me to believe we can beat HIV/AIDS, one child at a time.

Don Black, for returning.

Carol Blackman, for teaching me to ride and to get back on the horse—literally and figuratively.

John Bulger, for your probing interest and for making me feel that I belong.

Gabriel Byrne, for your friendship and for helping me face the crowd without having my knees wobble.

Kenneth Cole, for your great personal style, your fearlessness and your commitment to the cause.

Olivia Cox-Fill, for being such a goddess to me.

Sarah Davis, for your expert and loving care of Andiamo and Cookie.

Sarah Dickman, for relentlessly pursuing me, for believing I could write this book, for insisting that I do so and for your amazing support and faith during every step of the process. You are magnificent, Glitterscotch!

Ambassador Mark Dybul, for sharing your invaluable insight into the intricacies of the pandemic.

Nick Ellison, for your unparalleled expert guidance, encouragement and belief in an unknown writer.

Mary Fisher, for inspiring me from the beginning to rage against the disease.

Nick Fowler, for encouraging me to write the truth.

Kevin Frost (and all of amfAR, especially Dr. Matilde Krim), for pursuing the cure with relentless zeal.

The "Girls"—Laura Benko, Kelley Binder, Courtney Phibbs Boyd, Erin Leopold Brinley, Collette Bruce, Elizabeth England, Marie Gantz, Chase Gulden, Abbe Hail, Susie Henkel, Chandler

Hopkins, Shannon Grace Margaret Kelly, Logan Levkoff, Elizabeth ("Sally") Molsen, Gala Narezo, Leigh Oblinger, Beverly Pattenden, Kelly Renwick, Whitney Ross, Shauna Sang and Edie Silver Walker—for the life-sustaining force of your collective friendship, guidance and love at countless GNOs.

Jeremy Grayzel for your patient mentoring, leadership, brilliance and encouragement, and for giving me a chance to try to make a difference with my pen and my voice. And Joan L. Brown for your always wonderfully positive feedback and for lending your artistic talents to the battle. (And JJ, for making me smile.)

Peggy Henderson, for always championing my cause.

Jim Himes, for sharing existential truths in the nation's Capitol.

Sean and Donna Holmes, for being such wonderful cheerleaders and for making my dream of a house come true.

Tim Horn, for your magnificent mind and your limitless dedication.

Bob Ickes, for resetting the bar for my written words and for your exceptional, delightful, life-bolstering friendship.

Selden and Kit Illick, for your kindness and for helping me share my story with our community.

Jane Jennings, for always being there, especially in the ER, with strength, glamour, sound advice and laughter.

Landon Jones, for sharing the secrets of writing and for your encouragement.

Rob Mandolene, for helping me show my face to the world.

Jennifer Morton, for your giant heart and amazing grace, especially under pressure.

Cheryl Olsten, for bringing beauty, friendship and stability into my life at a time of great ugliness and uncertainty.

Pam Parson, for your loveliness—inside and out.

The indescribably talented and dedicated staff of POZ—present and past.

Bert Rinkel, for helping me to heal, and for taking away my fear.

Michael Sennott, for being my sage and for delivering God's love.

Happy and Sam Shipley, for your magnificent vim and vigor and for your loving support.

Keith Snyder, for your love—and your music.

Peter Staley, for your amazing counsel and support.

The incredible Laura Stern, for saving me from myself and for reassuring me, over and over, that I could write my way out of the abyss and into the light. Your graciousness and friendship, talent and sensitivity made one of the hardest years of my life worth every agony. Also, Emily Bestler, Judith Curr and the whole wonderful team at Atria Books, for making my dream of writing a book a reality.

Megan Strub, for sustaining the life force that is *POZ* and for your friendship.

Sean Strub, for creating *POZ*, for being such an incredible role model and for always pushing me to dig deeper.

Jody Suozzo, for resetting my compass. And Chris Tomalin, for being a light in my life.

Wolfgang Thom, for your divine presence.

Bryce Thompson and Grace White, for providing me with a safe shelter from the storm.

Lyerly Spongberg Tuck (and Daphne and Olivia), for reminding me to dance and wear sparkly things, especially when the days get dark. And Fred Tuck, for dancing.

Ann and Ramsey Vehslage, for supporting my journey.

Bill Wadman (and Cookie!), for the picture of the pretty horse.

Dr. Pelli Wheaton, for teaching me to live above the wound.

Paul Worley, for the soundtrack to success.

Also, the countless leaders and other people serving in the HIV community, whose passion and determination is an inspiration to me every day.

And, finally, each and every person living with and affected by HIV/AIDS around the world, especially those whom I've had the pleasure to meet, for driving me onward. You are why I can do what I do and why I will not stop until the stigma is gone and we find the love and compassion all people fighting illness deserve. The communal strength of your surviving and thriving despite the virus silences my complaints, dries my tears and re-ignites my fire to fight HIV/AIDS every single day until I die.